MY PTSD SOUL

MY PTSD SOUL

Taming the MONSTER under the bed

Annalise Green and
Earl E. Hocquard, MALLP

XULON ELITE

Xulon Press Elite
555 Winderley Pl, Suite 225
Maitland, FL 32751
407.339.4217
www.xulonpress.com

© 2024 by Annalise Green and Earl E. Hocquard, MALLP

All rights reserved solely by the author. The author guarantees all contents are original and do not infringe upon the legal rights of any other person or work. No part of this book may be reproduced in any form without the permission of the author.

Due to the changing nature of the Internet, if there are any web addresses, links, or URLs included in this manuscript, these may have been altered and may no longer be accessible. The views and opinions shared in this book belong solely to the author and do not necessarily reflect those of the publisher. The publisher therefore disclaims responsibility for the views or opinions expressed within the work.

Unless otherwise indicated, Scripture quotations

Paperback ISBN-13: 979-8-86850-590-4
eBook ISBN-13: 979-8-86850-591-1

[https://docs.google.com/document/d/1ngWy9FcTysNaHiD7abVp5FXA44khZtCholKilTwc2KU]

Dedication

This book is dedicated to all those affected by PTSD/CPTSD who have suffered in silence and are making that courageous journey to "get their lives back" and to those who have suffered and who have reclaimed their lives from "the monster under the bed." We hope the pages of this book, though not an exhaustive roadmap, will help you in your journey to grieve, address "the monster," and find hope and validation to begin to heal. Whether you are a member of the military, in law enforcement, or a civilian who has faced very real trauma, this book was written with you in mind.

Recommendations

"Easy to understand and challenging. I would call it a 'great tool book.'"

—Al Eldridge, 1st Sgt., retired U.S. Army

"In *My PTSD Soul*, Earl Hocquard instructs and informs the reader about post-traumatic stress disorder (PTSD) and its relative, complex posttraumatic stress disorder (CPTSD) in an easy-to-read and effective way. Earl's choice of co-authoring with his client—who has experienced PTSD—in the first several chapters was brilliant, as her eloquent journal entries paint a picture that gives Earl the ability to interpret and explain what was happening in her life. Also, that both coauthors have experienced PTSD and CPTSD adds a layer of authority as well as relatability to the book. Later, Earl shares practical helps to help the reader navigate their next steps in the healing process. Many will truly benefit from this insightful book."

—Barbara Arrabal-Hamper, MS, school psychology; PPSC, school psychology; former school psychologist in the Los Angeles Unified School District, Los Angeles, California

"In a society of positive thinking and the 'get over it' mentality, we have learned to deny grief and have encouraged others to bury their trauma, which is damaging to the very soul. Earl and Annalise do a beautiful job of encouraging us to face our monsters, and their book gives us the hope of living healthier and more realistically."

—Kelly Lynn, *Living Free Consulting*, BA
in secondary education

"I believe this book will help so many and encourage us all to embrace self-compassion! This book is brilliantly written with the key elements to healing oneself presented one step at a time. The deep dive into raw, vulnerable experience paired with timely compassionate language completely elevates self-awareness and understanding with words that describe exactly what is happening when trauma energy is in the mind and body. The book goes even further to then nudge the reader, with loads of encouragement and hope, to take the opportunity to practice how to move through and integrate trauma. While down to earth and full of clarity, this book is also spiritually uplifting. I recommend reading every page and journaling every prompt. It is worth your time and effort because *you* are worth your time and effort!"

—Danielle Stokely, LCSW

Contents

Introduction(s) xiii

Chapter 1 Broken 1

Chapter 2 The Movie in the Next Room................15

Chapter 3 Ants, Butterflies, and Speed 27

Chapter 4 Who Pulled the Trigger? 43

Chapter 5 Has Anyone Seen the Instruction Manual?....59

Chapter 6 Forward Movement and Containment........75

Chapter 7 Where to Begin?..........................97

Chapter 8 Practical Helps to Get the Kind of Life
    We Want: Understanding Our Brain and
    How It Works 105

Chapter 9 Practical Helps to Get the Kind of Life
    We Want: Proven Stress Relieving Exercises........111

Chapter 10 Practical Helps to Get the Kind of Life We
    Want: Helpful Processing 131

Chapter 11 Practical Helps to Get the Kind of Life We
    Want: Facing Giants, Beginning to Heal...........145

Conclusion 165

Author's Biographies...............................171

Introduction

(Annalise)

This is not a cookie-cutter how-to manual. Every struggle is different. If you are reading this to understand someone with PTSD, or you're experiencing it, or you're just interested, please keep an open mind. Everyone's story is as unique as the fingerprints we possess.

This is my experience. I hope it sheds light on the monster under the bed. You will read some excerpts from my journal entries. I didn't begin my journaling right after the incident. It took a couple years. I kept saying to my counselor, "I hate writing. I don't want to journal." Well, I finally picked up the pen.

So, let's get started.

Introduction

(Earl)

If you're reading this book, it's likely you or someone you love is suffering from PTSD, or post-traumatic stress disorder. A newer initialism is CPTSD, which is complex PTSD. The difference is that CPTSD is caused by a series of events over time that have been traumatic or an event that has happened over a long period of time.

Wait! I thought only soldiers got PTSD or CPTSD. Though our brave men and women in uniform can and do get PTSD or CPTSD, the disorder is not limited to the military or law enforcement. Civilians who witness serious trauma to others or who experience trauma themselves can develop PTSD/CPTSD as well, whether it's on foreign or domestic soil.

According to the *Diagnostic Statistical Manual of Mental Disorders, Fifth Edition (DSM-5)*, the symptoms that can occur with PTSD are the following:

- Experiencing a traumatic event(s)
- Witnessing a traumatic event(s)
- Experiencing repeated/extreme exposure to a traumatic event(s)
- Intrusive/distressing memories of a traumatic event(s)
- Recurring and distressing dreams/nightmares related to the trauma(s)

- Flashbacks that cause one to feel as if the trauma were actually happening in the moment
- Intense and prolonged psychological stress
- Marked psychological reactions
- Persistent avoidance of the stimuli associated with the traumatic event(s) (avoiding distressing memories, thoughts, feelings, people, places, conversations that are related to the trauma)
- Inability to remember aspects of the trauma (dissociative amnesia)
- Persistent and exaggerated negative beliefs regarding one's self, others, or the world
- Persistent negative emotional state (anger, guilt, shame, fear)
- Marked decreased interest in activities
- Feeling estranged or detached from others
- Persistent inability to experience positive emotions like loving, happy, and satisfying feelings
- Irritability and angry outbursts
- Reckless or self-destructive behaviors
- Hypervigilance
- A heightened startle response
- Difficulty with concentration
- Sleep disturbance

A quick disclaimer: If you are experiencing these symptoms, please see your doctor, a therapist, or a psychologist who can professionally assess and diagnose PTSD. Like many disorders, some symptoms of PTSD/CPTSD can overlap with other disorders. A number of symptoms must be observed to accurately diagnose and treat PTSD/CPTSD.

Introduction

My coauthor and I have suffered from PTSD, though in my case it was CPTSD. We know the reality, horror, and dysfunction that this disorder can and has caused in us and in others. We are deeply compassionate with fellow sufferers. Though my CPTSD has been in remission for about five years, I still deal with and feel the occasional triggers, fear, and anxiety. Thankfully, I'm able to navigate through it quicker today than I could in the past. The intensity is much less as well.

Though the *DSM-5* lumps PTSD with death or near-death experiences, I have personally seen several individuals who have had nondeath trauma—such as severe financial crisis, a traumatic divorce, or a traumatic loss of a job—that developed PTSD or CPTSD symptoms. These nondeath traumatic events deeply affected these people, and PTSD symptoms surfaced significantly in their lives.

Through reading the pages in our book, you will probably feel the "darkness," the despair, and the reality of PTSD/CPTSD. You will hopefully feel validated and that you are not alone. Also, we'll present some healthy and practical tools you can implement along the way that will help you slowly get your life back. Sure, the scar(s) will be there, but the "open wound" can be healed (though not forgotten) to a good degree. Taking this perspective, there's no pie-in-the-sky cliches, no "Christianese," and no "take two scripture passages and call me in the morning"–type approaches, only practical help.

Our prayer is that you will recover the puzzle pieces of your life to eventually not have to live in survival mode. The Savior who died a brutal death on a Roman cross and rose bodily from the dead is the same Savior who said to come to Him and He would give you rest. He gets it!

1

Broken

"What's wrong with me?" I asked my doctor. "Tell me what's going on," she said.

I went on to explain something like this:

"My eyebrows, eyelashes, and hair are falling out. My nails have stopped growing, and when they finally grow, there is this ridge at the base. I have this feeling like you get when you sit outside the principal's office—that jittery, nervous feeling with sweats, like you're in trouble. I have no appetite and exhausting mood swings. I stutter and I'm tongue-tied when I speak and can't seem to find the right words to say what I want to say. It's hard to hold conversations. I have a lack of focus. I'm wide awake at 3:00 a.m. I don't want to leave the house for fear."

"What's been going on in your life?" my doctor asked.

I shared what had happened. I began to tell her I had lost my husband several months prior in a boating incident. We were on vacation. I will not go into detail as they're not what is important. I will only say that I had to save someone else while I watched my husband drown because I could not get to him. When I finally was able to get to him it was too late; he slipped under the water just as I reached for him. Gone. I was left out in the middle of the ocean, holding on to a seat cushion while the man I saved helped another friend (he was struggling in the water, too). It was horrifying. Time stood still. It seemed like I was floating there forever, alone.

This was more than grief, she stated. She asked me if I had ever heard of PTSD. Of course I had; that's the thing that soldiers and victims of violent crime get. Oh, I was so ignorant. I wanted to get better and to be fixed. I was broken and wanted the pieces put back together. Could I be normal again? Was there a normal?

PTSD makes a person feel broken. Here are some excerpts from my journal discussing some of the areas that I feel are in pieces. They are not in chronological order.

The Defining Moment

October 30

I said something shortly after the incident that was a falsehood. I said with all my believing heart, "This is not going to define me." How utterly absurd! To think that such an event would not affect every aspect of my life was pure naïveté. My sleeping, my waking hours, my relationships, my expectations, my new marriage, my perspective of God, my entire being was affected. It *does* define me. I am who I am, right now, because of that event, PTSD and all. Even PTSD has brought a new definition to my life. Perception of myself and the world has changed. I don't see myself as a victim. I see God differently, too. I wish I could put my finger on it. At times it's more distant. And at other times, it's more humble and pleading for healing—never doubting His love for me, yet questioning the method of His workings. The pain for my children, the void that will always be there—the first grandchild, the weddings.

My spirit was and is so confused. I never doubted that that was his appointed day.

What I get angry and hurt over is that I had to witness it and be helpless to stop it. Why God allows something like this, knowing how absolutely crippling it can be, has been a question on my lips. I feel useless now. My mind gets fuddled up. My memory is shot. My word-find can disappear at times. My ability to handle circumstances that require multiple disciplines has been feeble. Some days I cannot make a decision without second-, third-, or fourth-guessing myself. Why would God, who wants the best for me, take me from a highly motivated, articulate, kind woman to someone who has difficulty going to the store to buy a gallon of milk or picking out the brand of toilet paper? (There *are* a lot of choices out there.) And don't ask me to go to Costco or Walmart. How is this useful for the kingdom? I don't see how any of this has been good. I just don't see the point. I thought I was a strong Christian. I suppose you don't see your weakness until you have been pushed to the breaking point. God broke me. I'm still in pieces. I don't know what the "fixed" me will look like. Maybe I'll be broken all my life. One thing is for sure: I'll never be the same."

****

First entry in my journal:

I can't even begin to explain how different my life is. It's been thirty months. I was a professor's wife. Small Christian college. When he got the position nearly a decade ago, I exited the full-time work scene and became a part-timer. Our kids liked that I was home more often. College life was packed full of obligations and responsibilities. The full, busy life with all our responsibilities left me drained. I was burnt out. I wanted out. Our life was exhausting. Scott wanted out, too. We wanted to do something different. We were looking at retirement in the not-too-distant future. We got what we wanted, just not as we expected.

There is so much to write about. Where to begin? God is a good place. I would fill this notebook with the complexity of His workings. I'm sure His hand will be seen as I write. How different is my life? I had reentered the full-time workforce. I was a CNA but decided to go for my EMT license. I like prehospital care. I was at a volunteer fire department and I worked for a few years before we moved for his new position. Except for my job now I have no continuity. Even my kids are ever changing and fluid. It's supposed to change as they grow up, but this was night and day. They had to grow up overnight, and I became a single parent. Nothing is the same. Absolutely nothing. As I lie here in a bed that's not mine, with a dog that wasn't mine, in a house that's not mine, I'm reeling from the facts of my life. *Is this really happening to me?* The facts that I face every day. Some component of *that* day invades my mind. I deal with it (not always well or in a healthy manner) and go about my day. How can I live within such flux? This transformation at my age. I can only handle each day. God has blessed me with a new husband, Luke, who nurtures me and caresses my soul; he lets me have those bad days. Understands me. What a treasure I have.

I have so many fears. Fears of pain, of loss, the unknown, failure, choices, people, Walmart, the night, passwords, salt water, lakes, oceans, and a plethora of other things. PTSD magnifies fear.

Last night our church small group was discussing Psalm 142. Our pastor preached on loneliness. Our leader asked us to share a moment when we felt the most alone. Instantly, I was transported back to that day while everyone was sharing. I was floating in that water again, grasping for Scott as he slipped under the water. He disappeared as the waves threw me side to side. I was lying across the cushion, screaming into the fierce wind—screaming, "Nooooooo!" over and over again. I have never felt so isolated and deserted by God. Psalm 88 was a reality. Even God had left me in my perception. The entire time that the others were speaking, I was having a silent panic attack, trying to hold it together as my heart was racing, palms were sweating, and skin was crawling. My flight instinct was almost unbearable. I wanted to bolt. I held it in and spoke when it was my turn. It was brief, very brief. Short and to the point. It was as if the oxygen had been sucked from the room. (This was the first time some of the group learned of my backstory.) Their faces said it all. I was trembling. A tear rolled down my cheek. Luke touched my arm. He knew those emotions. That empty place.

The nightmares continue. The insomnia is still there. I am weary.

****

I am exhausted after something like that. Retelling my experience, no matter how brief, saps all the energy out of me. Maintaining control is excruciating.

Journal Entry:

I don't dream sweet dreams anymore. No dreams where I smile, laugh, or fly. I loved dreaming of flying. Now I don't want to go to bed. I know what could await me.

November Journal Entry:

The nightmares have slowed down for now. But the panic and anxiety have resurfaced. I don't know which one I prefer. I think panic and anxiety. At least they don't leave me in a grieving state. No gut-wrenching sobs upon waking. No confusion or deep, deep sorrow and that soul-crushing fear of loss. No, I really think I prefer the panic. Those ants are easier to tame than the grim reaper in my dreams.

****

Part of being broken is the dreams that torment you. My sleep is broken. Nightmares come in bunches. Sometimes it's about death, usually the death of someone I love. Sometimes it's just spiders crawling all over me or a killer chasing me. I am crying, screaming, or whimpering, and Luke has to bring me to an awakened state as he holds me. Then I sob in his arms. Other times, I awake and know I was having a nightmare but cannot recall the dream, just the horrible emotions that have left me sweaty and feeling terribly sad. My teeth hurt from clenching my jaw. I hope my sleep returns to normal someday.

The Emotion Thief

Journal Entry:

Spent the first night in the new house. Too many months since I slept in my bed. Forgot how firm it is. Slept poorly: new house, new sounds, new smells. Luke and his kids moved most of the big stuff in as I worked yesterday. I was having a bad day.

I said nothing to them when I got home. No "thank you" was said by me. I had no joy or sadness about this. This hurt Luke. He didn't understand my lack of emotions. We were finally in our home, the one we built together, but it didn't mean anything to me at that moment. That is something PTSD has done to me. It steals emotions. Sometimes I'm overly emotional, making me cry, panic, or super joyous. Then the thief comes. It brings apathy and a coldness. I have nothing. It's like you used up everything in your tank and you're on empty. It's all wrapped up in turmoil, guilt, and anger. (You know you should feel something, but when you don't, you have guilt.) So, either the feelings flood or ebb as a drought. And the people closest to you watch this rollercoaster ride. They think you are unstable or losing your mind. *You* think you are losing your grip, too. They also may feel that you are angry with them, as Luke felt tonight. So, both parties watch this trainwreck and feel helpless. And I feel guilt. I always feel guilt.

****

The Unbalanced World

Jan. 12. Journal Entry:

I'm greatly fearful of loss. Like getting bit by a dog as a child makes you leery of all dogs, I'm petrified of loss. I handle it poorly. I cushion myself from thinking about it. Unfortunately, the event has me in a state of rumination. I love so many people, especially my family, that the thought of losing anyone again sends me into a tailspin. How do I balance it? PTSD takes my world out of balance. Vertigo. I've had vertigo twice. The first time, I didn't realize it had come upon me. I awoke and got out of bed or at least tried. I felt strange. The walls were moving, and I couldn't stand. I immediately fell to the ground. (*Am I having a stroke?* came to my mind.) Then, I felt the typical spinning, and nausea followed. Even crawling to the bathroom wasn't in a straight line. I have never felt my body so uncoordinated or my sense of reality askew. I tried to stand. I couldn't. I grasped for the walls for fear that the floor was going to shift from under me. My rationale knew that the walls and floor were stationary, but all my senses were screaming something different. My mind and body were out of sync. I wanted the floor to have handles. It was a helpless feeling. No one could have convinced me that the floor wasn't moving. PTSD gave me spiritual vertigo. My mind said, "God loves me," but my heart and soul were breaking and felt utterly unloved.

****

Being broken comes in all forms: anger, irritability, fear, depression, sobbing, edginess, and a whole list that I can't even come up with right now. People who are broken desperately want to be fixed, but no one told me, nor did I guess, it would continue as long as it has.

Feb. Journal Entry:

Three years ago a coworker lost someone to a car accident. That was the beginning of a chain of events in my mind, terrible events full of sorrow and loss. Soon my three-year event marker will be coming upon me—hard to believe. I wonder sometimes if I am depressed. *Would I even know?* I have little drive to do anything. Some days I can go from zero to sixty and back to zero. Some days I have energy to walk, clean, grocery shop, and work, but most days I don't want to get out of my chair. I haven't taken my anxiety med for two nights. Unfortunately, I've slept poorly. I don't want to have to have them. I fear that I will become dependent on them. Looking back on my life, there were times when I knew I was in a state of depression. However, I believed it would have been frowned upon to seek medical help or therapy. It's a struggle to want to get better because you *know* there is something on the other side yet you'll never pursue it because of the stigma attached to it.

As Christians, we need to look differently at people who experience depression or who suffer with PTSD. We didn't choose to be in this traumatic event. It has wounded us, is scarring us, has left us breathless and shattered our world. I want to be normal again. I want the memories erased. I've heard many preachers say something to this effect: "You're depressed? Complaining? Find somebody to serve. Stop being so selfish or self-focused. This will fix you." I used to somewhat agree with this attitude until I actually experienced depression, anxiety, panic, deep sorrow, and PTSD. I've *never* felt sorry for myself. I've *never* called myself a victim. There have been many selfless people who have been thrust into a pit they didn't dig. This was me. This is me. Don't tell me to "just get over it." I'm not fixed yet.

I've noticed that my digestive issues flare up with increased anxiety. This is a new symptom. It has morphed. I said to Luke that I thought I was getting better. I became irritated with myself. Apparently this is a chronic thing. I was blindsided again with all of this.

****

Since that journal entry, I have discussed with my doctor the depression I have had through the years. It has gotten pretty bad lately. I sit in my chair and stare or cry for long periods of time. I sleep for long periods, have no energy, and always seem to be on the verge of sobbing. I am now on antidepressants. I don't feel shame that I asked for something. It's a tool to help me get over the hump. After all, I have to admit to myself that what happened to me *was* traumatic and horrible. No shame in that.

The way I see it, there are three types of people out there when you are in a pit:

You have the one at the top, looking down, telling you to get over it and get yourself out of that hole.

The second type is the person reaching down trying to pull you out and cheerleading you on. They have great intentions, but the pit is much deeper than their reach.

The third type will get the tools and equipment needed and jump into the pit with you. Together you build the ladder to slowly climb out. The third one takes time, effort, compassion, and just enough sergeant-like attitude to not let you give up.

When your world has come crashing down, you want to gain control anyway possible.

Journal Entry:

OCD. I see this in my life as I have had to declutter and downsize. I had to purge my belongings and sell my house—my beautiful house; 90 percent of the "junk" was my late husband's. He kept everything. I was frantic to purge, clear out, downsize, minimize. I never liked all the stuff. Now it rested squarely on my shoulders. I was angry. More than angry—pissed! *How could he leave such a mess for me?* It overwhelmed me. It took nearly three years to go through his stuff and get the house on the market. It was a monumental task. It was emotionally excruciating and exhausting. I jumped in and started sorting right after the memorial. It gave me something to do and occupied my mind. I now have an ever-growing aversion to clutter and nonessential items. It's almost to the point that too many belongings make me twitchy. I suppose it's because I *never* want to sort through thirty-five years of memories again. Anger would build within me. The responsibility fell to me.

Clutter makes me feel like chaos has taken over. I can't control my life, but by golly, I can control how many pizza cutters, vegetable peelers, coffee mugs, old chargers, old computers, old phones we have and to what compass position the forks are pointing in the tray! I want to plan out everything. Shouldn't I rely on God to direct my path? This is dangerous. He has sent me down a rough road. My trust is shaken. I've seen His blessing and provision, but I've also seen the fire. It scares me. It scares the crap out of me. I'm afraid He will do it again. The pain, that is.

My trek didn't start this way. I didn't know it would lead to the haunted forest. If God put me on this path that led to this event, then I'm not so sure I want to trust Him. It sounds absurd. The God who died for me is hard to trust? Well, yes. I can't control Him. He's not a tame lion. I'm not writing heresy. He knows my emotions, my struggles, and innermost questions. I'm just being honest with myself. I look at the Psalms. The psalmist lays bare his soul. Trying to pretend that I didn't/don't question Him would be a lie. My soul is in conflict. The PTSD triggers are sneaky, like a lioness crouched in the tall grass. Yup, there's a spiritual battle of trusting God after something like this. He has no obligation to tell me why. He's God. I'm awestruck by His love, yet terrified by His ways.

What's Happening Here?

(Earl)

Annalise uses some very good words and a word picture to share what the experience of PTSD was and is like for her. Those who have or who have had PTSD can definitely resonate with what she wrote.

Let's take a quick peek at some of her language here to describe her monster under the bed. Annalise writes, "My rationale knew that the walls and the floor were stationary, but all my senses were screaming something different. No one could have convinced me that the floor wasn't moving."

This physical symptom of vertigo is an excellent example of what PTSD does to an individual emotionally. As Annalise said, "PTSD gave me spiritual vertigo." PTSD gives us an image, thoughts, feelings of being right there in the trauma as if it's happening right here and right now! Many times we know we're in the present and not back in the trauma; however, the emotions of fear and the fight, flight, or freeze response feel as if the trauma were right here in the present. We can see the trauma happening in our mind's eye. This image is like a bowling ball, and our rationale is like the pins that are knocked down by the image and the thoughts and feelings of dread and fear. It's a perfect strike but one that we don't want.

I remember about maybe six years ago I was in a meeting. The individual who was speaking at the time made an innocent comment. It wasn't wrong, but it was a comment that triggered my PTSD. All of a sudden, I felt intense fear. I knew I was in the present and not back in the trauma; however, like the vertigo Annalise talked about, emotionally I felt like I was there! I felt fear and nervousness, had flashbacks, and the flight mode kicked in and I wanted to bolt out of there! I had feelings of not belonging in that meeting because it triggered my PTSD!

Annalise continued and said, "My mind said, 'God loves me.' My heart and soul were breaking and felt utterly unloved."

In the song "The Wreck of the Edmund Fitzgerald," Gordon Lightfoot penned the lyrics, "Does anyone know where the love of God goes when the waves turn the minutes to hours?" As believers we know the love of God goes nowhere. His love is with us. With this, we don't feel it all the time with PTSD. We question it. We search for something we feel is not there. We ask ourselves, *How can a loving God let this happen?* This is the haunting question that bombards our mind with no answer. At this moment, the PTSD sufferer doesn't need correction, a sermon, or advice. The sufferer simply needs a listening ear and a caring heart that understands why the question is being asked. They are processing an event—a trauma—that makes no sense to them. It's therapeutic to talk. That's why we call it "talk therapy." Allow them to talk without judgment.

Annalise writes, "People who are broken desperately want to be fixed, but no one told me, nor did I guess, it would continue as long as it has."

It's like the femur bone. It's the strongest bone in our body. It's a critical part of our ability to move and stand. In other words, it's important! If this bone is broken or shattered, it's not going to be a quick fix and easy recovery, though we would love for it to be. It's going to take surgery, a cast, many months, possibly rehabilitation, and many small steps with setbacks before one is able to get back to normal activity. This is what Annalise came to know.

Many mean well. Many of our fellow brothers and sisters in Christ mean well. With this, it's not helpful to expect or demand quick recovery from someone with PTSD or CPTSD. "Just look on the bright side" isn't going to cut it. "Here's a verse you need to hold on to" isn't a magic pill. "Let go and let God" comments will shame the sufferer into feeling they aren't doing enough. Why? Because the brain is a computer that stores information and memories. It does so to inform us and protect us from future traumas. *Apparently, you need to do more,* the brain tells us. Yes, there's good help. With this, it's not immediate.

Annalise authentically says, "I was pissed!"

This connects to something else she said: "There have been many selfless people who have been thrust into a pit they didn't dig."

Yes. This produces anger. It *wasn't* fair. We didn't ask for this. Plus, anger is a natural and normal expression of grief. One of PTSD's symptoms is irritability and anger. The unfairness of life and the grief of the trauma produces anger. What Annalise was feeling was as normal as breathing. I applaud her honesty and the courage it took to share her real feelings.

Later in our book we'll look at things that can and are proven to help with PTSD/CPTSD. For now, let's normalize the feelings that sufferers go through.

2

The Movie in the Next Room

[*Static needed.*]

"Stop! Just stop it!" This is what I tell my mind. Trying to escape your own mind is impossible. So, what have I done? [*Static.*] Google defines TV static thusly: "Noise, in analog video and television, is a random dot pixel pattern of static displayed when no transmission signal is obtained by the antenna receiver of television sets and other display devices." To the younger generation, this is gibberish. However, we older people know what that means. It is an interruption of signal to our TV show. We got to watch black, gray, and white dots with that irritating buzz of "ssshhh." This is what I have looked for. I desire the static. I want the signal to be disrupted.

March 24 Journal Entry:

Been having some sadness lately. Don't know where it stems from. I just want to be held. Tears are nearly always on the brim of my eyes. Again, I feel raw. Exposed. That's the best description of my emotional state. I want fresh, new skin, or maybe calloused so things don't make me bleed so easily. I've been able to listen to more Christian music lately without it affecting me as it once did. Those songs should bring great joy and praise but instead I would be crushed. This baffles me. Aren't Christian songs supposed to uplift us believers? Instead, it brings loss and *that* day. All emotions, all fears, all sadnesses, all anger, all frustrations, all panic comes from that day. How do I get away from my own thought processes? Staying busy helps. Facing them is supposed to be helpful. Sometimes, I face them and the battle is won. Sometimes, I choose to pull the covers up and hide my face. Either way, it's always there, that movie playing in the other room. Maybe progress is slow, maybe I am getting better. Maybe it just takes a long time. Damn it, it's taking too long.

****

[*Static Please.*]

January 14 Journal Entry:

Why do I feel the need to have my Air Pods in my ear, listening to music, a constant hum of sound? I don't really like the TV on—can't stand commercials. But the Air Pod is soothing. It's not loud. Does this give my mind the stimulation I want or need? Does it cover up my overthinking and analyzing of thoughts, white noise for the mind? I can even hold conversations while I have one in. Sometimes I have slept with it going. Got it going even now. Before the incident I would have not tolerated it. Now I seem to crave the static. It keeps my mind from going to *that* day. Strange: I have changed. Many things about me have changed. I guess I really won't ever be the same. It's a puzzle to me.

****

The Movie in the Next Room

The best way I can describe this thing that your mind does to you is like a movie in the next room. It's the same movie playing over and over (the incident). It's not really loud, nor are you watching it all the time. It's just there, always running in the next room. You know it's playing because you catch a couple scenes or familiar lines from the actors. You try desperately to block the signal by creating your own static. Sometimes it works, sometimes it doesn't and you have to endure a scene. The movie never stops. You can get away from it for a while, but you know it's always going to be there. In time, you move it to the farthest room and stay on the other side of the house. You learn to build a larger house so there is a greater distance between you and it. Sadly, it's still running. I realize that it will always be playing. I can never get away from those memories. I want to buy a ticket for a different show. Making new, great, happy memories has helped.

I spoke about keeping busy. Busy sometimes doesn't work.

Distractions

April 14 Journal Entry:

Been painting the new house. I'm much calmer during these periods of projects. Luke saw it when I had to paint my basement for the sale of my house. It staves off panic and seems therapeutic. Why? Whatever the reason, it works. But I can't run on a project-driven, busy-centered life. That's not reality. I guess the new house, selling the old house, finishing the quilts, moving during the holidays, and setting up a new household is my new big project. I literally started feeling panic rise within me as I wrote those tasks down. Ugh! A list of tasks incites a tightening of my shoulders, elevates my heart rate, and brings a feeling of an adrenaline dump with those butterflies. So why do I run toward them? To keep the movie from becoming too loud? I find that the list is the problem, not the actual tasks. Funny, huh?

It's a fine line between static and solitude. I crave both.

Solitude vs. Static

January 6 Journal Entry:

Noise. Quietness. Which one? I really like quietness in the morning. Luke prefers the TV in the morning. Everyone is different. I could go days without TV. There's something about TV that can get on my nerves. Some people like the background activity and conversations. I, on the other hand, feel as if the people on TV have invaded my personal space. Is that what I feel when I enter one of those huge, busy chain stores? Why does it ruffle me? Interaction with people drains me. It can be exhausting. So much emotional energy just to be with people. I even felt this way before the incident. After a few hours with people, I was wiped out. Sometimes, even friends are draining. God created us to live in community. I guess I prefer small community. I feel I wasn't cut out to be a professor's wife. I should have been a farmer. I do better with animals. I find it easy to disconnect from people—not my family, just others. (I'm not saying that I don't or didn't love them.) Animals are calming. They're simple, not complicated. They're not pretentious, nor do they have ulterior motives. I'll take people in small doses.

****

Anonymity

I stopped going to church all the time. Some people passed judgment on me for this. They didn't get it. I was mad at God. When I did want God, I didn't want to share God with anyone. I didn't want to be distracted by others. I wanted to cry whenever I wanted. I didn't want people to look at me in pity. I didn't want to talk to them. Words were meaningless. They didn't know anything of my pain. My best friends became strangers. I was a stranger to myself. How could I be a good friend when I had no emotional energy for them? I wasn't being self-focused. It was just exhausting to go out of the house. I knew they loved me. The energy it took just to be in a group was draining.

When I returned to church, I found a place where I wasn't known, a place where there were no memories. Anonymity was a wonderful gift. I could be alone in a crowd. No responsibility to them. I didn't have to converse with them. This sounds so cold and heartless. It was survival. It was a time to heal. I was using all my energy to keep it together. I had none left over. I didn't want to be known. I wanted to be invisible. Sometimes I wanted to be invisible from God. For God to view straight through my soul can make me uneasy when I don't even know what's in there. Maybe if He would have just forgotten about me, He would have done something different that day. Isn't that silly?

Continuing my Journal Entry:

A question for my counselor: Do people like me feel a disconnect from their former life? This brings me to cheesecake. I love cheesecake. Just the mention of it brings the taste to mind. That tanginess, that smooth texture, the sweet fruit topping. Yum. I liken this life-disconnect to a lost recipe. A strange memory. Something that I can taste in my mind but will never have the actual thing again. All cheesecake will have a different taste from now on. They will all have different ingredients. Almost like I *never* ate that former recipe. I will never experience my old life again, just strange memories that seem surreal. I can't explain it. It's as if I have two lives in my head. If I didn't have children, I would think it was an apparition. Almost as if thirty-five years didn't happen. Except for those intrusive images of that day, I would believe it to be a work of fiction. Damn images! Is this normal? I hope not. I want to be normal again. Maybe I am normal. My new normal.

Everyone is broken. Just some of us hold more pieces in our hands.

****

Dogs are great.

June 2 Journal Entry:

It's been a week since I have recovered from influenza B. I lost my sense of taste and smell. Good thing, too. I had an ambulance request for a dead body and an elderly female that needed transport to the ER. This one shook me. It's been a while since a call has affected me like this. It was a very elderly couple. She has severe dementia; he took care of her. He died suddenly, right in front of her. She was in her chair. She had been there for nearly two days. He was lying on the floor in front of her. She was nonambulatory. It struck me tonight why that call flustered me sorely. I can't imagine what had been going through her mind. I know what was going through my mind as I watched Scott die. Maybe dementia was a blessing today. I wish I could forget what I saw.

I need to talk to Earl, but our availability doesn't jive. Glad to have my dog. I was sitting on the floor of my shower, letting the water flow over me. I had it as hot as I could stand it. Wanted to wash off everything from the day. Luke is traveling again for work, so I have no one to talk to. (He's usually in flight, so I can't even call him.) So, I sat there, sobbing again. I find myself in this place often. My sweet doggie, who hates water, pushed the curtain aside and stepped right into the shower stream. He was getting soaked. I was sitting there, legs bent and knees drawn up, my forehead resting on my knees with my arms wrapped around my legs. Water was falling, and my body was shaking from the force of my sobs. He started to whine. He came closer, started licking my arms and nudging my legs. We both just sat there, me sobbing and him sopping wet. I stayed there until the hot water ran out, forcing me to get out of the shower. It was ugly, very ugly. What would I do without my dog?

****

Additional thoughts:

The movie will always play in my head. Sometimes I don't notice it. Learning to accept this truth has helped me tame it. It will always be there, somewhere in the background. May I never forget the preciousness of life and the brevity of it. This should make me a better person.

What's Happening Here?

(Earl)

Let's dissect Annalise's journaling and see what's going on in her life with the presence of PTSD. Annalise writes, "Either way, it's always there; that movie playing in the other room. It's just there, always running in the next room. In time, you move it to the farthest room and stay on the other side of the house. I desire static. I want the signal to be disrupted." This refers to the thoughts of the trauma. This refers also to the flashbacks of the traumatic event—the "movie" and the "characters" and the "scene" that keeps playing on repeat that she so desperately wishes would shut off or end. Even on better days, the movie can be heard "just down the hall" as a TV show can be heard a few rooms over.

Why is this? The trauma was real. It wasn't an "unfortunate event." It wasn't "God's trying to teach something." It wasn't that she picked door number one but should have picked door number three. No. The trauma was real; therefore, the present *movie* is real.

We can see the avoidance of the movie as well by moving it "to the farthest room." People experiencing PTSD/CPTSD desperately avoid the thoughts, conversations, people, scenery, or anything else that reminds them of the trauma because it surfaces those feelings that scare the soul out of them, so to speak. This is a symptom of PTSD. It's a normal survival mode the brain uses to keep the fear and anxiety of the trauma at bay. This is good and needed… for a season. Eventually, it's healthy and needed to slowly move toward those thoughts, conversations, people, and scenery to begin to accept and start to heal and get our lives back.

Annalise said, "This movie will always play in my head. Sometimes I don't notice it. Learning to accept this truth has helped me tame it." We'll look at this later in our book. For now, we're looking at the normalcy of all this.

Annalise goes on, "A question for my counselor: Do people like me feel a disconnect from their former life?"

Quick answer is yes. Why? Annalise answers this in her comment: "those intrusive images of that day."

Again, our brain "disconnects us" from "that day." It's too painful. It causes too much anxiety. It hurts too much. It's too uncomfortable. It's too (fill in the blank). Our brain protects us. Again, this is good and needed for a season; then, it's good and needed to start to face it with a trained counselor who can walk us through the memory of the trauma.

Annalise continues, "Been having some sadness lately. Don't know where it stems from."

Again, Annalise answers her question by penning the word *exposed*. Trauma *exposes* us, wounds us, causes very vulnerable feelings, and shows us just how susceptible we are as human beings. (This is not a putdown but a validation of our reality.) This will cause depression and sadness and grief. It's as normal as a Michigan 85-degree day in July.

Do you notice the events of trying to soothe the pain in Annalise's journal? "The Air Pod is soothing. It's not loud. Does this give my mind the stimulation I want or need? Does it cover up my overthinking and analyzing of thoughts?"

The answer is yes and yes. It's both soothing *and* it covers up. The healthy middle ground here would be the balance of self-soothing *and* starting to address the trauma.

Annalise shares, "Sometimes, I face them and the battle is won."

There is an element of withdrawing in PTSD/CPTSD. Healthy? Unhealthy? Let's see how Annalise frames it. "Aren't

Christian songs supposed to uplift us believers? Instead, it brings loss and *that* day. I stopped going to church all the time. Some people passed judgment on me for this. It was survival."

There is a part of withdrawing that I wrote about in my book (coauthored with Carl Hamper) *Healing the Wounded Spirit*, where I said that moments of withdrawing are and can be healthy. Withdrawing allows us the space and time to feel our grief and to mourn it without all the other-imposed mental gymnastics. If we're *always* around others, we don't get the space and time to mourn—*unless* we are specifically around them to grieve/mourn and gain support. Being around others constantly is a "filler" and can prolong the grieving process. Hence, Annalise cut back on her church attendance to have that sacred space to be alone with her thoughts and grief and to conserve her energy. Plus, happy songs (of worship) can bring feelings of shame to us. It's not that the songs themselves or God produces shame; it's the notion that *everyone else seems happy… and I'm not*. Or, *I'm supposed to be happy… and I'm not*. Hence, the retreat of some of her church attendance.

I remember a period of three months (several different times) during my CPTSD that I refrained from going to church services. The mental gymnastics were too much for me to bear. I didn't "quit on God." I just refrained from going to church services for a season. It proved to be a great and fruitful season of some healing for me.

The pastor at that time was including degrading remarks in his sermons. I'm sure he didn't mean to; however, they were less-than-helpful remarks. He would say, for about a month straight, "If you do it God's way He'll bless you to death! If you do it God's way, He'll bless your socks off!" My problem was that *I did it God's way*, and the trauma that changed my life happened anyway. It wasn't God's fault; it's just that God's not Santa Claus, who always brings us goodies when we're good. Life is real, and life hurts at times. It doesn't mean we did anything wrong! Another more hurtful comment was when he (the pastor) would tell the congregation that people would come up to him and say (then he changed his voice to a whiny voice), "Pastor, I'm hurting. What do I do?" Then he would answer the question in a demanding voice and say, "You trust God! Can you say amen, church!" That was the straw that broke the camel's back! I had to stop coming for a season. One of the best three months of my life!

What if a woman who had been raped recently was listening to that sermon? Or a parent who had lost their child in an auto accident? Or a spouse whose partner died of cancer at thirty-nine years old? Or a mother whose son was sentenced to ten years of prison? Or a physically abused person? Or _____ (fill in the blank)? Do we see how it benefits others and ourselves to use some compassion, tact, and wisdom here?

Annalise goes on to write about a little light at the end of her tunnel. She writes, "Making new, great, happy memories has helped." Awesome! Notice how she didn't claim that all old traumatic memories have disappeared. It's because they didn't. They're still there. With this, new, great, happy memories are simply added.

I've heard it put this way: Trauma is like a blacktop being laid for a road. The trauma "paves a road" in our brain. It's real. It's there. All other thoughts "travel on that road," and that's why we have the fear and apprehension and hypervigilance we do. When we intentionally add, as Annalise said, new, great, happy memories from good experiences, they begin to pave over the top of the trauma road in our brain. Eventually, that's the road our thoughts travel on. Make no mistake, the trauma road is underneath; however, the new road is paved over the top, and that new memory becomes the new road our thoughts travel on, though we are aware of the road underneath. The brain is quite remarkable.

3
Ants, Butterflies, and Speed

Hold on for the ride.

The monster brings exaggerated emotions, adrenaline dumps, and terrible energy. Now I understand why people go off their medications to experience a manic episode. I never felt so alive and young. I miss the endless endurance and activity. I don't understand why this happens. I'll just share some of my journal entries and be transparent. I don't like to be vulnerable. Sharing with you makes me uneasy. It's not an easy thing to open up.

November 14 Journal Entry:

Need to discuss something with Earl. My manic period. Lasted about a year. It started sometime between Thanksgiving and Christmas. I began to experience a manic state of mind and body. At least that's the best description I can come up with. I had decided to decorate for Christmas. I bought a four-foot, tabletop tree. It was lovely. I figured out how to put it together by myself and actually enjoyed seeing it there in my dining room. I cried a bunch while doing it, but I did it, nonetheless. I wanted some Christmas decorations for myself and my children.

I was trying to maintain some normalcy for this first holiday season without him.

By this time, my appetite had virtually disappeared. I had begun to lose weight, for which I was elated. I had been struggling with middle-aged pudge for a few years. I was also enjoying the freedom of not being at a Christian college, the life in which every minute seemed to be filled with responsibilities and obligations. We weren't just a professor and wife, we were shepherds, like other staff. No praise team practice, Christmas parties or programs, costume design and sewing or such. The busy-ness of Christmas was left behind. Anyway, I was enjoying my independence. I got my younger shapeliness back, and some gentlemen friends had expressed their interest. (I was not ready for any relationship.) I was not held down by church or scholastic commitments during this time. It had just been an overwhelming responsibility. I could travel if I wanted or relax.

For the next several months I found myself in a state of abundant energy, creativeness, sharpness, heightened senses, verbally articulate (as well as written), with an optimistic outlook and an ever-growing desire for the new and unknown experiences. For lack of a better term, I think I felt how someone having a manic episode might feel. I survived on little sleep and sustenance. I found myself painting my kitchen at 4:00 a.m., cleaning up, and going to work for a twenty-four-hour shift. I increased my hours at work. My kids must have thought I had lost my mind. I wasn't home much, and when I was, cleaning, sorting, purging, painting, and whatnot were performed. I had the exuberance of a teenager with the thirst for life to match.

Rewind a little. At one point in November (several months after the accident), I decided that I was "gonna live!" God didn't take me that day, so there's living to be done! This was pivotal. It didn't stop the crying or the grief, fill the huge hole in my heart, or end the loneliness or the anger. It just put a different lens to my spectacles. This manic state was a gift. I believe it gave me the energy and drive to keep going during a crucial moment in time.

It was during this time that I met my current husband. He'd lost his wife nearly a decade before. We had some mutual friends. We met for coffee and grief support. A friendship started, but that love story is for another time. Back to this mountaintop attitude…

I ventured out and sought another church. The one that my late husband and I had attended was becoming increasingly painful to enter. I was only going for one of my kids. My other children had already left. They could no longer endure the pain that the memories invoked. Scott had been an elder, and we were involved in nearly every ministry there, too. Well, back to the mountain…

On this mountain, I learned to be self-sufficient and found myself. (Who *I* was without Scott.) I was married for nearly thirty-five years. I never knew adulthood without him. I had also been diagnosed with PTSD. What a conflicting time. I felt most alive when all the while I was experiencing the depths of immense sadness and grief combined with anxiety attacks, invincible and dreadfully scary. Needless to say, I felt unstable but wonderful in the same twenty-four hours. Heck, in the same twenty-four minutes! I thought PTSD was for soldiers. I had no idea that I could have this condition, one that brings scoffs and eyerolls and carries strange connotations and is shrouded in questions. I didn't understand myself; how could I understand what was going on with me?

One time—I was having a perfectly good day—I pulled into Sam's parking lot to do some grocery shopping. I began to shake and sob uncontrollably. Luke had to text me through the episode. (I was unable to talk to him.) I was there an hour before I could go in. But I did go in. That was not an isolated incident for Sam's or other large stores. Sometimes, I didn't make it in to go shopping. I don't go there alone. I switched to a smaller grocery store where there are fewer people. Apparently, these large stores are a universal trigger for us PTSDers. Triggers? I didn't even know there was such a thing. I was so ignorant. So what was happening to me? I cannot say.

Being a woman of faith, I would lean toward a strength from the Lord. Such a magnified sense of life. As I stated, during this period of manic energy, I had keen senses and the ability to have a heightened awareness of all my senses. Everything was crisper, more tangible. I could describe the "smell of green." My mind seemed to combine colors with thoughts and my olfactory sense. Poetry flowed, and descriptive language was easy. I felt as if my creative IQ had risen fifty points. Unfortunately, my ability to make decisions and be alone were at rock bottom. My mind raced all the time. I had spent months and months after his death sorting out the financial aspects of our life. To this day, I'm still dealing with areas of it. I was exhausted from making decisions. I didn't even want to choose what brand of shampoo to buy. It was all too overwhelming. Tedious, repetitive, frustrating was everyday life. The amount of times I had to tell somebody that I needed to change the name of the billing statement because my husband died was a marathon. Frequently, they didn't get it right. It had no end. I relived the event every time. Wham! Slap in the face when the mail came. I still carry

Ants, Butterflies, and Speed

a death certificate in my car (over three years later). I'm going to need it again.

Sometimes, I long for those days to return, the manic days. It almost felt like I was on some kind of drug. Mind you, I've never used drugs, but I've seen their effects. Is this strange? I don't know. (The more I experience life, the more I realize that I don't know much.) The appetite has returned, along with the pounds, minus a few. The heightened senses have backed off. Superhuman energy and stamina have ebbed, but so have the frequent sobbing outbursts.

I still experience anxiety. There are different kinds: crowd, choice, password, alone, water, whatever. I've learned to live with it. Living with it is like playing football and you're the quarterback. You know that you will be sacked some time during the game. However, you play anyway. You have to. Unfortunately, it's when I get blindsided that ruffles my feathers. *Wham!* Out of nowhere comes that three-hundred-pound defensive lineman. A good scenario is the one where you get clobbered, lose a few yards, but get back up to continue the game. Some plays you lose more yardage than others. The best days are when the pass is complete. I choose to play like it's first and ten.

Now, if I can just get rid of those ten extra pounds.

****

Some additional thoughts I would like to share:

During this time, I challenged myself to overcome some fears, tested my better judgement, and looked for adventure. I did some stupid things that won't be mentioned. I forced myself to climb the scaffolding and paint my vaulted ceiling and walls (approximately fourteen feet high). This may not sound like a scary thing to some, but to me it was terrifying. I don't like heights. I couldn't do this years earlier when we were building the house. I rode my motorcycle too fast and traveled alone. I craved that feeling of being alive and a little frightened. I wanted to prove to myself that I could do things by myself. I wanted to be self-sufficient. With the exaggerated emotions came extreme highs and desperate lows. Sometimes the Emotion Thief knocked and apathy entered. I wanted to feel something! I wanted to be alive because I felt dead inside. I wanted out of that empty. The only way out was to be frightened or overstimulated. I became an adrenaline junkie.

I also began to drink. I liked the way it challenged the Emotion Thief. I was changed into a giddy and carefree person. It took the empty and filled it with something. It's a poor way to cope or escape. It's not sustainable because it's a false happy. Some people drink to numb the pain, while others drink because it makes them feel good. Either way, it's a lie. Unfortunately, I still resort to it sometimes. It's a short escape. During those moments, I don't care if I know it's a lie.

Trying to Outrun Anxiety

August 10 Journal Entry:

A list of tasks incites a tightening of my shoulders, elevates my heart rate, and brings the adrenaline dump with those butterfly vibrations. This is how I would describe it. "Hello, my old companion. It's been a few days since we've talked. I would like to instruct you on your behavior while in my house. However, you burst in unannounced and disrespect my rules. I will try to ignore you as you follow me around the kitchen, shadowing me so close I can feel your nasty breath on my neck. At some

Ants, Butterflies, and Speed

point you will either leave quietly or bring me to tears and anger. You will steal my thought patterns, patience, words, rationale, joy, my neat and tidy world. You disrupt everything. You are the worst houseguest. I would demand that you exit, but that scarcely works. Some days I can outpace you. (The busier I am, the harder it is for you to keep up). You do seem to find that backdoor and sneak in. I could move, find a new town or life, but you always find me."

So I stand my ground and face it. The Lord gives me strength. That day is a victory. On that note, some days I feel like He has lost sight of me and my struggle. I know He hasn't. It just feels that way. I wish my feelings could be tethered by my faith. I know all the right methodology and Bible-speak to accommodate that statement. Too bad it's not that easy when your body, emotions, and mental faculties declare mutiny against your faith and rationale. Lock and load; here comes the fight.

****

This chapter is titled "Ants, Butterflies, and Speed" because of the physical symptoms I experience. I have many times felt as if there were ants crawling on my skin and the desire to bolt to escape the present situation. I feel this way when I am in a crowd. Before the incident I could tolerate crowds fairly well. It wasn't my favorite thing in the world, but it didn't bother me. Now, I become physically uncomfortable. My skin crawls sometimes. I fidget. I constantly tap my foot, rub my fingers, flip my hair, and so on. I become uncomfortable in any position I sit. My shoulders become so tense. I constantly have knots in my back and neck due to this. Skin tingles and crawls. I become super sensitive to noises and even the texture of my clothing.

My PTSD Soul

It is as if I have ants on me. The only relief is when I am alone. This is a double-edged sword.

The butterflies are the physical symptoms of the heart palpitations and that general feeling of all my body quivering or jittery. Too much caffeine? It's hard to explain. It's butterflies all over. This is more of an inside-the-body feeling. It's that wonderful butterfly feeling in your stomach when you kissed your first love. It's amazing! Well, it's amazing during that short ten seconds. Can you imagine that feeling for hours or days? It becomes your enemy. It drains you. It makes you jumpy and an insomniac. You are constantly trying to slow everything down so you can get some sleep. Your heart races and skips beats for no apparent reason. Your insides can't stop moving. You just can't stop.

Speed. Speed is in my mind. It's that racing. Maybe a normal mind has a slow, meandering, Sunday afternoon ride kind of thing going on. Not mine. I can never turn it off or slow it down. Remember when I mentioned the thing about the movie in the next room? It's something like that, only it's not about the incident. Not only is the movie always playing, a bazillion other items are running through my head. My husband says that there's chaos up there. He has no idea. I am bombarded with the things I have to do, things that might happen, things that are happening. I constantly think about the small scratch on the wall that needs to be touched up, the hard water spots on the faucets, the stock market, the children, that shirt that has to be mended, car needing an oil change, bills to be paid, the friends from ten years ago that I have lost contact with, and so on and so on. I look at my sweet dog and wonder about the day I will have to say goodbye. I see in my mind's eye the funeral of my children, my parents, my new husband. My mind races in all directions. I am hijacked by this locomotive. I wasn't like this before. I had my usual concerns and worries but nothing like this. I am no longer the conductor. The train is a runaway and I can't get off. Speed.

As you can imagine, this is exhausting. You are physically tired but never sleepy. Your mind is on a kamikaze mission. I felt supercharged and focused, but I wasn't focused on the right things. I was a battery that was overheating and didn't even know it. I couldn't continue like this. As much as I liked many aspects of this, I had the realization that someday, like the battery and kamikaze pilot, I would crash and burn.

What's Happening Here?

(Earl)

I wish Annalise wasn't such a good writer; this way my comments would be brief. However, since she is fabulous, I must comment more in length. (My apologies.)

Annalise writes in various places in this chapter, "The monster brings exaggerated emotions." "I found myself in a state of abundant energy…" She felt "dreadfully scared." "It was all too overwhelming." For her, "frustrating was everyday life." "With the exaggerated emotions came extreme highs and desperate lows." "I felt dead inside." "I was trying to maintain some normalcy…" "It didn't stop the crying, the grief, fill the huge hole in my heart, or end the loneliness or the anger." "Triggers? I didn't even know there was such a thing." "I wish my feelings could be tethered by my faith." "It makes you jumpy."

Excellent descriptions, Annalise!

Can we see the various emotions/turmoil/experiences that were going on in Annalise? Wow! High energy, fear, feeling overwhelmed, frustration. Also, there were extreme highs and desperate lows, feeling dead inside, outbursts of crying, grief, emptiness, loneliness, and anger. There were triggers (or events that sparked the thoughts and feelings of her trauma) and then feeling jumpy (or on edge or nervous). Her faith in God didn't even tether her feelings/emotions. We see hypervigilance sprinkled in here, possibly feelings of a high startle response, numbness, and desperately trying to grasp for some normalcy. Again, all of these are very normal symptoms expected with PTSD/CPTSD.

As I mentioned earlier, we'll explore things that will help us on our way toward healing later in our book. For now, I want to focus on the normalcy of what Annalise and others were and are feeling and experiencing. It's very important to validate what's felt and experienced before we look at things that will help.

Annalise writes, "I survived on little sleep." Also, "my appetite had virtually disappeared."

This speaks of depression, which has various symptoms. These can be two of them. Now, some who are depressed can experience a lot of sleeping and an increased appetite, way more than usual. Others can experience very little sleep and barely have any appetite. People respond differently. When I had my CPTSD, my sleep totally changed. I used to take naps, slept deeply when I slept, and could sleep ten hours. After my CPTSD, I rarely, if ever, take naps. I sleep lightly, and I can wake up in the night or wee hours of the morning and can't go back to sleep. This is still the case, and I've been in remission around five years. I get a good seven hours; even with this, it's not the same as it was. (I'm sure age affects this, too.)

Ants, Butterflies, and Speed

When one has PTSD/CPTSD, they are "grasping for straws"! What I mean is that they are seeking relief. I fully understand. Annalise wrote that she began to drink. The pull toward alcohol, drugs (prescription, too), sex, food, and other distractions is or can be strong. As Annalise alluded to, it's only a temporary fix. These are unhealthy vices we can get ourselves in. Now we not only have PTSD/CPTSD, but there's an addiction that causes health problems, strained relationships, and it can stunt the healing process. I get the pull. With this, if we desire healing way more than burying the trauma, this helps us begin to do the healthy things for our bodies, our relationships, and our mental health.

Annalise recalls, "It was during this time I ventured out and sought another church. The one that my late husband and I had attended was becoming increasingly painful to enter." "I switched to a smaller grocery store where there are few people." Here we see "downsizing" and change due to pain, memories, and the flight response. Now, what do we do? Do we make changes or "stay in our present situation"? Both. Huh? Both. It depends on what the change is. I'd work with a trained therapist in PTSD/CPTSD to determine what to change and what to wait on changing. Some changes may be needed sooner than later and other changes later than sooner. It would be impossible to list them here. That's why I'd recommend a trained therapist to help guide the process. In Annalise's case, I think that changing churches and "downsizing" to a smaller grocery store was the right change she needed. It helped to foster a little bit of healing.

Annalise so beautifully described the "brain fog" that can accompany PTSD/CPTSD. She wrote, "Your body, emotions, and mental faculties declare mutiny against your faith and rationale." (Keep in mind the word *rationale*.) "You will steal... my rationale...." "things that might happen..." "I am hijacked by the locomotive."

Regarding the amygdala, Daniel Goleman writes in his book, *Emotional Intelligence Why It Can Matter More Than IQ*, "When it sounds an alarm of, say fear, it sends urgent messages to every major part of the brain: it triggers the secretion of the body's fight-or-flight hormones, mobilizes the centers for movement and activates the cardiovascular system, the muscles, and the gut. Other circuits from the amygdala signal the secretion of emergency dollops of the hormone norepinephrine to heighten the reactivity of key brain areas, including those that make the senses more alert, in effect setting the brain on edge" (page 16).

Goleman uses the term throughout his book. It affects our rationale/logic. In this definition we can see the fear, fight, flight, freeze, and hypervigilance response of the brain. In short, though Daniel Goleman can describe it way better than I, picture our brain as an aircraft (a plane). The prefrontal cortex, which is the logical, problem-solving part of the brain, is the "pilot." The amygdala is the "hijacker" in the back of the plane. The amygdala alerts us of danger. So when the amygdala says, "Warning," the hijacker makes its way to the "cockpit" and hijacks the prefrontal cortex, or the logical and problem-solving part of the brain, and takes over. This greatly diminishes our ability to think more clearly and logically.

Going back to Annalise's "rationale difficulty," this is why. The amygdala hijacked the logical, problem-solving part of the brain. In this case, the hijacker (or amygdala) can pretty much take the plane (or our thoughts, which create emotions) pretty much anywhere. Hence, anxiety, fear, and the worst-case scenario, panic, overwhelm. At this time, though we may know we are not back in the trauma, our emotions indicate that we are. It becomes an emotional flashback.

I remember I had the privilege of facilitating a veterans support group for a year or so. One class we were sort of talking in small groups and I heard a vet say to another vet, "Do you hear that?" I hadn't heard anything, and I have good hearing. All of a sudden, I heard a helicopter fly overhead. This vet, who flew in helicopters in the Marines, heard the sound before I did. He was hypervigilant (aware) because of what he'd been through. The amygdala put him on alert.

Experts with the brain who are way smarter than I have said that the brain cannot distinguish between real threat and perceived threat. Threat is threat. The body can go into fight, flight, or freeze mode with the announcement that one's company they work for is laying off a number of employees indefinitely—even when they don't know it'll be them who will get laid off. The brain sees perceived threat as threat, too.

We'll get more into this later in the book. For now, we can see what's going on in the brain during these triggers that cause fear or intense fear.

Listen to Annalise: "I constantly think about the small scratch on the wall that needs to be touched up, the hard water spots on the faucets, the stock market, the children, that shirt that has to be mended." "I fidget. I constantly tap my foot, rub my fingers, flip my hair, and so on."

Annalise also alluded to a tight back, neck, and shoulders, as well as heart palpitations and decreased sleep. These are what we refer to as psychosomatic symptoms or physical symptoms brought on by emotional and psychological pain. Here we see anxiety, hypervigilance, and, due to these, a need to try to control her outer world. Annalise couldn't control life and the hard hits that life threw her way. However, she could control the scratch on the wall, the water spots on the faucets, and that shirt that needed to be mended. Those of us with PTSD/CPTSD try desperately to control our outer world because we can control the little things, like Annalise wrote about. There's an element of healing in this. Controlling comforts, and it slowly builds our confidence. Along with this, it's imperative to keep this in balance—to be intentional—about what we are doing and why we are doing it. The reason is if it gets out of balance, we train our brain that "being a control freak breeds comfort and healing." But when it's in excess it doesn't. It breeds more angst and anxiety and irritability because we cannot control everything and everyone, though we subconsciously try. Control little things, not the world.

Annalise said, "I challenged myself to overcome some fears, tested my better judgment and looked for adventure." "So I stand my ground and face it. The Lord gives me strength." Yes! There comes a point when more healing and getting our life back more comes with doing what Annalise said—facing or exposing ourselves to the difficulties. In therapy we call this "Exposure Therapy." We'll go more into detail later. For those of us who are believers, the Lord *is with us* in the pain, struggle, and journey as we navigate through PTSD/CPTSD.

Allow me a moment to share something that seems counterintuitive. It's called "facing it, embracing the pain, entering the traumatic memory, grieving the loss." This sounds counterintuitive because everything within us feels it's *good* to do the *opposite*.

Recently I got vertigo. Never had it before. Horrible! Woke up with my room literally spinning like a ceiling fan for a matter of what felt like minutes. Afterwards, I had bouts of severe to mild dizziness. As I write this, I'm still in the process of recovery.

There's this treatment called the Epley maneuver that was administered to me on more than one occasion. Worked great! Plus, I have to do eye and neck exercises to help with balance. However, the "trick" is that I had to be willing and intentional to willfully *make myself* dizzy—cause the room to spin like a ceiling fan—in order for the treatment to work. *Whoa! What?* Everything in me yelled, "This isn't a good thing!" However, it *is*. I had to "bring on" the symptoms in order to navigate and come out the other side nondizzy.

It's the same with our emotional pain, our trauma, our traumatic memories. We want to *not* give them any space, thinking that they will eventually go away. They don't. They just get buried. Like the Epley, we do well to enter into them, give them sacred space, and "make ourselves dizzy" so that we can eventually come out the other end more healed. Yes, it sounds counterintuitive. I get it. Trust me, it's *not*.

Annalise recalls, "I had no idea that I could have this condition" (PTSD). "One that brings scoffs and eyerolls and carries strange connotations and is shrouded in questions."

It's sad that we can scoff at what we don't understand. I remember losing my mom. We were close. Because I dealt with grief and some depression over it, I got "the third degree" from some. I got "a sermon" of what *I wasn't* because I grieved. Mind you, by this time I was an orphan with no brothers and sisters. I was alone. Those who reprimanded me had siblings *and* both parents still living and healthy. If you're reading this to understand a loved one with PTSD/CPTSD, please don't scoff at what you may not understand. A safe relationship is the best therapy for PTSD/CPTSD per Linda Graham, MFT.

Annalise vulnerably and wisely said, "The more I experience life, the more I realize that I don't know much." (This doesn't have much to do with PTSD; however, it is awesome and wise to adhere to!)

Thanks, Annalise, for painting a masterpiece of what PTSD/CPTSD looks like.

4
Who Pulled the Trigger?

Triggers. What? What are Triggers?

Puking Dog

January 12 Journal Entry:

Sometimes my anxiety comes like a puking dog. *ROOOHHG, ROOOHHG, ROOHHG.* I can see what's going to happen. I run to the door and call the dog, hollering, "Nooooo! Nooooo!" Too late. A pile of dog yack on the rug. Yup. I holler at myself in my mind. "No, no, not here, don't do it!" Too late. Pile of yack.

****

Blindsided

Sometimes something that you never saw coming will rattle you. Blindsided. You are defenseless. It comes from the blind spot.

May 3 Journal Entry:

Sat here and sobbed. Tonight I feel alone. Desperately alone. Luke travels for work so he is gone again. I have felt this way before. When I was alone, floating on the water. I don't know why the emptiness flooded over me. It was heavy. Nearly tangible. Again, being alone is scary, but being with people can be overwhelming. Places are scary, too many people are exhausting, usernames and passwords are terrifying, and being alone can be desolate. Today I had a bad panic attack. It was out of the blue. Wham! I got in my car and immediately knew that someone had been in there. Gloves were disturbed. The garbage from the little can was on the floor. The water bottle was on the floor. I didn't get upset as I'm not paranoid. There was a good explanation, I was sure of it. I tried to ask Luke about it, but he was unavailable. I texted him and asked him to call me. I started off to church. On the way, I started to sweat, my heart rate became rapid, and an overwhelming feeling of being violated came over me. Someone had been in my car. It took me about an hour or so to calm down. My shirt was soaked, and I was exhausted.

I finally was able to speak to Luke. It was him. Before he left for work, he put up my windows because it was raining, and the water bottle fell into the garbage. All that fuss over something simple. I kept trying to tell myself that it wasn't anything to get upset over, but my body had other plans. Why did the thought that someone had been in my car send me to the edge and push me over? I don't know. I wish I did. My reaction bothered me as much as the thought of someone in my car. That feeling of an invasion into my personal space. *My* car. This car has not been shared by my kids or husband. Exclusively mine. It sent me into fear. Vulnerability. Danger. Exposed. Threatened. Like I said, I'm not paranoid, but this shook me.

I guess since the accident, I want every place that's mine to be safe. My car became scary. Places aren't safe.

Who Pulled the Trigger?

****

The Safe Place

January 8 Journal Entry:

"I don't have a place," stated Stacey as we sat side by side on the stairs. Holding her face in her hands, she was crying. We were moving her out of her home. Life had changed for her, too. She was having a day of memories, and emotions flooded over her. One of our close friends was sitting at his mom's bedside, waiting for her to pass. This brought back a load of heavy memories for Stacey. Memories that were less than a year old. She had sat by her mom's side, too. She had no place to retreat to. The familiar has been ripped from both of us. That got me thinking. Where is my place? That spot I go for solitude.

I moved into Luke's house after we got married. It was not *my* house. I didn't belong. It was small, old, and in the city. I disliked it, really disliked it. I found myself going to the furnace room. It was warm but devoid of sunlight and had been set up as a sewing room for me. However, it still wasn't mine. At my house my place was my bedroom. I had a huge bedroom with windows that extended from floor to ceiling, a French door that led to a balcony, a chair, a side table, and abundant sunlight. I looked out over a small depression of trees. We had a large home in the woods. I would peer into the treetops, hear the birds, and enjoy my refuge. I allowed the emotions to flow. I would retreat there often after the accident. The ugly, plaid chair embraced me while facing southwest. The sunlight poured into that room. It was the most beautiful thing. I could see the glass needed a good cleaning. Old bottles of various, mismatched colors stood in the transom. The light made them give up their hues. Standing there, they seemed to be looking down on me like little protective soldiers as tears gathered then streamed down my cheeks. I relish the sunlight. It made them unique. The imperfections of old glass. Air bubbles. Dirty. Weathered. Beauty. A reminder of my childhood.

We would go from one old farm estate sale to another looking for these gems. I love antiques and looking for the grandeur in each old farmhouse, the outbuildings, and stately red barn. That's where generations past would birth children, raise hard workers, and eat dinner at five o'clock. It was my dad's passion. I got the love for old things from him. Simpler times. Bottles just make me smile. I could say that we're all like bottles. Imperfect, dirty, chipped, cracked, full of bug skeletons and dead spiders that someone has to clean out. When I allow God to shine through me, I have a unique beauty. Wow. That sounds so cliché. I just rolled my eyes as I wrote that. But in all seriousness, it's not the clean, perfect, or boring cookie-cutter person who gets to experience the depths of God. That place, where I felt safe, is where my guard is laid down. I can expose myself to the healer. Luke's house doesn't have that. It's a depressing house. I will work on finding a place.

****

June 24 Journal Entry:

When I would see my old friends, they would say, "I miss you."

I would often reply, "I miss me, too." I didn't have anything else to say to them. How could I tell them that I am not the person they once knew, the person who could be the alpha, the strong one, the one who held people and gave courage and encouragement, the one with answers, with suggestions, with purpose and poise? I was demolished. I was left in a heap. Scott's death changed me. Remember that statement I referred to just a week after the incident? "This won't define me!" I was so defiant when I said it. So confident, yet so ignorant. I was in a state of denial and shock. I thought I was strong enough to push through without it changing me. Yeah, I miss me, too.

****

March 18 Journal Entry:

Friends are exhausting. It is too difficult to keep in touch with old friends. I had changed. The relationship had changed. Everything had changed. It was easier for a while to forget about or just not pursue or have friends. When I was with friends, I had to expend a great deal of energy to keep my composure. To be upbeat, courageous, and friendly. Almost like a facade. Many times I didn't want to be exuberant or open. I did not want to speak to anybody. I wanted nothing to do with places. Places scare me. What if I had a panic attack or something was encountered that triggered a memory and caused pain? *Maybe a small, unoccupied cafe?* No, even those are too unpredictable. Remember, places are scary. I didn't want to spend extended periods of time with people.

Conversations were clumsy at best. My thought patterns were fragmented, and my word-find was frustrating. Several times I thought I had dementia. Attention span was gone. I had no interest in anything. I could not hold a thought in a streamlined fashion as everything was jumbled in my head and it was racing at a hundred miles an hour.

Once I began to cope and manage my monster better, I stepped out into the friendship realm. I started to make new friends. These new people hadn't known the old me. That was liberating. They weren't expecting anything different than what they saw presently. I'm not saying that I don't miss my old friendships. It's just that I don't know how to be their friend anymore. I was also their shepherd in many ways. I didn't want that responsibility. It was and is too weighty for me. So, there is this heavy guilt on my shoulders. Being with them brings back so many memories. Then the pain of the loss, the guilt that I couldn't save him, and the shame that I have lost the desire to connect with them floods my heart. God is still paving new paths and friends. Forward movement looks different to everybody. I will never be the same, and therefore I'm scared that I will never be the same type of friend.

****

When I started to see what triggered me, I would avoid those offenses. I guarded myself from situations. Of course this would add another edginess to my life. Walking around with a protection plan in hand became my goal. Because really, who wants to see a grown woman have a meltdown? Not me. Unfortunately, I cannot protect myself from life. I learned that the triggers morphed. It wasn't just the sight of water or the smell of the ocean that made me sweat any longer. It was secondary remembrances, something that caught me off guard, things that reminded me of the entire situation. That day, that week, and the circumstances that were left for me to deal with.

Who Pulled the Trigger?

March 21 Journal Entry:

Another bad dream last night. It didn't have Scott in it, however. It had spiders. I'm not afraid of spiders or mice, but when they are crawling on you when you're in a confined space, it can feel pretty scary. So this is the third nightmare this week. What fears do I have lurking underneath? What has triggered these? I just want to be held. I fear being alone. Some nights, like this one, I desperately need to be held and it's not an option. Luke is traveling again for work. I sobbed for an hour. It isn't grief anymore (I think). It's just too many raw emotions. So few people understand the struggle. I want to be held, but no one is here. I have the fear that Luke will stop loving me. I'm fearful that his love is waning. I just want this day to be over. Why can't I gain stability again? I want off this rollercoaster. I feel thirteen again. It sucks.

****

Don't make me choose anything.

December 16 Journal Entry:

Before the accident, I could handle a multitasker's dream to-do list. Now, just thinking about a list sends me into a black hole. I second-, third-, and fourth-guess myself. I run from decisions. I want someone else to step up. Part of my traumatic event was about a decision. I often go through the scenarios but come up with the same or worse conclusion. That nasty, little ankle biter thought creeps in: "If only." The "if onlys" suck life out of people. So now, I don't want to make any decisions providing an avenue to screw up. Deferring to someone else takes the responsibility off me. Which brings me to that point: responsibility. Before, I could handle that backpack slung over my shoulder. Now I leave it on the floor, giving it a wide berth. I avoid it like a bad mother avoids a poopy diaper. *Let someone else have that gem.* So why do I react that way? I don't want to make the wrong choice again. I feel that I made a mistake and it cost Scott his life. It is my fault. I robbed my children of their father. There, I said it. I don't ever want to make another mistake. It takes too much energy to be responsible. When all your energy is sucked out of you as you muster up the strength to go get a dozen eggs, you have nothing left for decisions. Your gas tank is on E. It's protection.

****

The Unexpected Breakdown

February 10 Journal Entry:

We have a three-day training going on. I have a sinus infection. On meds. Still need to go to class. I feel horrible. Todd taught about diving emergencies. Had to leave for part of it. Underwater images set me off. When he got to the drowning portion, I couldn't take it. Luke was texting me through it. I tried to be strong. Obviously, I am not. When I got home that evening, I thought I was doing well—that is, until I became irritated. It's the furniture. I hate it. The living room is too small for all of it. This new house is a downsize to be sure. I tried to find my decor to make me feel at home. Rummaged through box after box. Couldn't find it. I want my old bottles. I want my house back. I wanted us to move into my house. I had a gut-wrenching sob. This continued for about thirty minutes. I changed the living room around four times. *Still not right.*

This was just the realization that I don't have another house to go back to. The old house will be gone on Monday. Somebody else's. Tomorrow will be the last time I step into *my* home. It makes me sad. Very sad and angry that I had to move away from my home because of this accident, this roller coaster ride. Hold on. I haven't sobbed like that in a long time. I felt grief and sorrow like I did after the accident. Everything upset me. I was irrationally angry. I had such seething rage. What did I take it out on? The *fridge magnets*. Fridge magnets and the stuff on the side of the fridge is something I despise! I hate it. I was so mad. I ripped everything off the fridge, throwing it across the room and screaming like a mad woman. The dog scurried away thinking he was in trouble. It's clutter. Clutter sets me off. I look forward to a place to put all this shit. The night never got better. I continued to scream and throw things on and off until I finally landed as a heap in my chair. I sat there, staring off into some distant memory. I was glad Luke was working again. I didn't want him to see me like this. I took something to help me sleep. I just want order.

****

Something I didn't understand was why I would have a trigger from something not directly related to the incident. I call them secondary triggers. Don't know if that is an appropriate term but I'm going to use it. Some of my secondary triggers came from the subsequent days, weeks, and months following the incident. The tasks that fell to me and the business of death. When I talk about the business of death, I am referring to the things I had to deal with. Name changes, bills, usernames and passwords that I didn't have and certainly didn't know, titles, insurances, house and car repairs, and so on. Each time I had to deal with those things, it became a frustrating nightmare. Over and over, calling people, telling people why I didn't have the correct password. I begged my late husband to write down all his usernames and passwords. He refused. He didn't think we needed a book full of them. I was trying to take the steering wheel of my life from a past that wouldn't let go. So, now when I have to set up an account somewhere and do the username and password thingy, I begin to feel that familiar quickened heart rate, sweats, butterflies, agitation, tears coming to my eyes, and the need to bolt. I feel overwhelmed. This wasn't me before the incident. Doing those things brings back the terrible memories, frustrations, anger, sorrow, and mental exhaustion that surrounded the accident. It isn't the actual accident; it was the struggle afterward. The triggers started to morph, and so did some of my signs and symptoms.

Death of Those I Love

November 26 Journal Entry:

Been many deaths this month. Angie, Grandma Linda, Pat's grandpa, Uncle Spence. Last Friday I had nearly an entire day of anxiety. I began my day with intrusive images. They came at me with ferocious intensity. I haven't had a day this bad in a while. I had chest pain, tightness in the throat, sweaty, rapid heart rate, all the classic signs. It was terrible. I had the same symptoms about a week prior too. On my way to work, a song came on the radio. I was triggered. I didn't tell Luke. He's been gone three days, and I didn't want to bother him. Maybe all these deaths and his absence has something to do with it.

Whatever the case, it was uncomfortable to be in my skin that day. I didn't have the emotional overflow that used to accompany it, just the physical symptoms. Next time I recognize it I will take half a Xanax.

****

The Unexpected Attack

December 31 Journal Entry:

New Year's Eve. Goodbye, old year! It's been a good year on some fronts. Thankful for all the good stuff. But today, today I really didn't want to do my job anymore. I had a sudden panic attack while driving to the hospital. It was on one of those roads that passes by the bay. There's a long curve that hugs it. It was pouring rain and cold. Roads and visibility were not optimal. Thoughts of slipping into the bay with the ambulance, water rushing into the compartments, sinking, drowning, disappearing came rushing into my mind. I nearly started screaming. Tears streamed down my cheeks, and I wanted to park the rig and go home. Well, that was impossible to do with a partner and a patient in the back. It passed, but it surprised me. That movie had never played in my head before. It was about that time that I didn't want to do this anymore. This hasn't been a problem before. I've never had these types of intrusive images. What triggered this one? Will there be more of these in the future? Sometimes there's no answers. I just want answers.

****

What are intrusive images, you ask? Well, it's like flashes of scenes from a movie. They come quickly, not in chronological order or in any organized fashion. They are blips from the photos in your mind of a particular event. Think of a happy day in your life. Wedding. Graduation. The new bike. Picnic. Birth of a child. The day you realized you loved that special person. The day you got that puppy. These are stored within your mind along with the emotion you felt that day. You can still smell the grass and wildflowers. The wind in your face on that carnival ride. It's all so good. Now, instead of all the warm fuzzies, you experience all the negative emotions. Fear, gut-wrenching sorrow, disbelief, guilt, confusion come at you for hours or days at a time. It's an overload. It wreaks havoc. It triggers panic.

Additional comments: Since writing these entries, I have left emergency medical services. I have had additional images like that one break into my mind. My husband's business is doing well enough to allow me to work part-time at a small gift shop. Nothing fast-paced. Easy going and little stress. I'm blessed to have this choice.

What's Happening Here?

(Earl)

Annalise put us in the driver's seat of her experience. Wow! What a wild and scary ride! Imagine how it felt to her. This is what compassion and sensitivity are: putting ourselves in another's experience and understanding what it must have been like. You see, we can be someone's healing by just being that therapeutic relationship. No, some might not be a trained psychologist or counselor; however, they can still help provide significant healing by being that therapeutic relationship that's understanding and safe. Never underestimate what can be done.

What weight to her words: "I miss me, too." "I thought I was strong enough to push through without it changing me." Trauma has a way of confronting us like that bully in grade school: confident, scary, big, and able to beat the snot out of us. Trauma humbles us and shows us just how human and fragile we are. That doesn't mean we're weaklings. No. It's just that strong people are *always* human and fragile when hit by trauma. Notice that I didn't say *God has a way of humbling us and showing us how human and fragile we are*. No. God is *for us* (Rom. 8:31 NIV). God doesn't need to do that. Sure, He counsels us. With this, we've taught people wrong that "God's gonna get us as His children!" There's enough stuff in life that will "get us." God already "got Jesus" on the cross for our punishment. God *doesn't* need to "get us"!

Let's look at Annalise's comments that come from a place of depression. "I had no interest in anything." "So, there is this heavy guilt on my shoulders." "I sobbed for an hour." "I second-, third-, and fourth-guess myself." "I became irritated." "My thought patterns were fragmented." "It was and is too difficult to keep in touch with old friends." These are all symptoms of depression (which can come with grief, too). Again, this is a normal occurrence with PTSD/CPTSD. It sure doesn't feel good; however, it is to be expected.

Let's look at Annalise's grief. "I just want order." "I had such seething rage. What did I take it out on? *Fridge magnets*." "Very sad and angry that I had to move away from my home." "The familiar has been ripped from both of us." These are thoughts and feelings of grieving. Anger is a part of grief. Again, normal.

I like what Annalise did—she tore into her fridge magnets when she was so angry! When we are angry, irritated, or grieving with PTSD/CPTSD, there are two extremes we want to avoid. One is exploding on others. The second is stuffing. If we explode on others, we ruin relationships. If we stuff we set ourselves up for more depression, which comes from anger turned inward. I wish I had realized this early on. I exploded—not in abuse but in making my wife feel on edge a lot of the time. So, beat up some "fridge magnets" or scream into or beat up your pillow. Maybe it's drawing angry faces or writing raw emotions in your journal with no judgment of feelings. It could be venting to a trusted and safe friend. Possibly doing as many push-ups as possible. Go for a drive and yell to God about what's making you so angry. Afterward, take some slow, deep breaths to calm. We'll go over this more toward the end of our book.

How about anxiety? Sometimes flashbacks accompany anxiety, or the other way around. Listen: "I began my day with intrusive thoughts." "So why do I react that way? I don't want to make the wrong choice again." "Underwater images set me off." "Another bad dream last night." Also, "So this is the third nightmare this week."

Bargaining is another stage of grief. There's denial, anger, bargaining, depression, and acceptance. These are like floors in a big building. We're on the elevator, and it will stop at random floors with little to no warning. We can visit the same floor various times. Annalise said, "I often go through the scenarios but come up with the same or worse conclusion." "If only." *If only I had left work when it was still daylight, I wouldn't have been raped. If only I left ten minutes earlier, I would have avoided that accident. If only I had said I loved them before they left. If only I had _____* (fill in the blank). We've all probably been

Who Pulled the Trigger?

there in some scenario where we said, "If only!" The guilt and the shame haunt us. Yes, there is deep grief in PTSD/CPTSD. With grief comes bargaining. We're trying to make sense of it all. Remember, in many situations, we made the best decision we could or that we knew at the time. Was it wrong? Was it right? Maybe it was neither. Maybe our decision simply *just was*.

What about those nightmares? Yikes! Nightmares can come in the form of the actual trauma. Raw and real! A fair amount of the time dreams and nightmares can come in the form of symbols as well. It's not a nightmare of the trauma itself; however, it can be something scary that is a symbol of the trauma, like Annalise dreaming about spiders crawling on her. I remember a recurring dream I had for ten years about three to four nights a week. A grizzly bear was after me to attack and maul me. If it wasn't a grizzly bear, it was a tornado. If it wasn't a tornado, it was a plane crashing in the near distance and me seeing and hearing the explosion. This was for ten years or more! These were symbols of a trauma I experienced.

FYI. I remember reading a psychology article that said if you're having recurring dreams and being chased by something scary, and in your dream you know it's a dream, stop and ask what is chasing you *who* or *what* it is. I did this with the grizzly bear ready to pounce on me. In my dream, the grizzly bear shrank down to what it was in real life. It was *me as a child*. In my recurring dream, I was being chased all this time by my childhood trauma. Funny thing, after that, I barely ever have dreams of grizzly bears or tornados or planes crashing. As they say, "If you name it, you can tame it." Of course, depending on the severity of the trauma, it may take longer to "tame it."

We're damaged goods, or so we feel. Listen to Annalise's glimpse of faith and hope: "When I allow God to shine through me, I have a unique beauty. But in all seriousness, it's not the clean, perfect, or boring cookie-cutter person who gets to experience the depths of God. That place, where I felt safe, is where my guard is laid down. I can expose myself to the healer." "God is still…" God is still what? God is still love. God is still present. God is still all powerful. God is still safe with us and our PTSD/CPTSD. God is still nonjudgmental. God is still gentle. God is still whispering to us. God is still fighting for us. God is still understanding. God is still…. Being thankful for this, and for the little things, brings another measure of healing.

Annalise pens, "It's been a good year on some fronts. Thankful for all the good stuff."

Yes, Annalise. This doesn't invalidate our trauma. It just says that life still has some good in it for us, too. Practicing gratitude and noticing the helpfulness of others gives us PTSDers more of a balance in how we view the world.

5

Has Anyone Seen the Instruction Manual?

Manuals are a great resource for people seeking to learn something. Have you ever tried to put together a bike, a kitchen faucet, or a Lego Star Wars Millennium Falcon without one? Don't you wish life came with a manual? I wanted one after the accident. I was older (a little beyond middle-aged) and thought I had my poop in a group. Yeah, it was quite a wakeup call to rise one morning with everything different. I remember the first few mornings after the accident. I had finally fallen asleep on the couch. I awoke to the crusty residue left by my salty tears. I was disoriented. When I gathered my bearings and remembered why I was on the couch instead of in my bed, I would start to sob again. I just couldn't get my mind around it.

April 1 Journal Entry:

A failed test. That is what it feels like. A test I could never study for. A textbook that was never written and a teacher that won't exist. I failed this test, and there is no way to redeem myself. I feel that I robbed my children of their father. Those thoughts flood over me often. Survivor's guilt? I sometimes feel that my children would have been better off if I had died that day instead.

My PTSD Soul

****

December 13 Journal Entry:

People love to tell you how to live. Suggestions fly thick like mosquitos in Alaska. Christians will say things like this:

You gotta just get closer to God.
Pray more.
Stop focusing on yourself.
Read your Bible more.
Get involved in God's work.
Pray harder.
Praise more.
Focus on His goodness and get over it.
PUSH. Pray Until Something Happens.
FROG. Fully Rely On God.
Let go and Let God.
Pray more and longer.
You shouldn't be on medication.
You're supposed to be relying on God for this.

Dollar store decor cannot be the mantra on which we hang the philosophy of our lives. Life is messier than a platitude plaque made in China. What most Christians don't realize is that even when all those suggestions have been instituted, PTSD is still the monster under the bed. And that monster scares the heck out of you because you have seen it. It's real, and even worse, it travels with you. It doesn't stay under the bed. I relive certain aspects from that week every day. The accident, the wind and waves, the aftermath, the police, the rescue boats, hearing "Mayday, mayday! Man in the water," the water, the phone calls, the faces of my children, the memorial, the voices, the cries for help, the weather, the smell of water, the messiness of death, and everything else that revisits me.

****

Believing It Couldn't Happen to You

July 17 Journal Entry:

Health, wealth, and prosperity doctrine. That's a bunch of bullshit. However, did I ignorantly, subconsciously think that terrible things couldn't happen to our family because we are good people? No, I wasn't living with my head in the sand. Nevertheless, it was a question that popped in my mind. Trying to make sense of it all. No one is guaranteed a good life. We are not spared from heartache. It makes us all the more aware of the frailty we possess—or that possesses us. We break easily. We bruise. We hastily cling to our tinfoil shield and raise it against the dragon. Only too soon to find our protection melts away under the brimstone breath. Some things we cannot control or protect ourselves from. Had I been lulled with the American attitude that heartache only happens to others? Mudslides in Central America destroying entire villages, tsunamis, murder, earthquakes, genocide were not waiting for me. No. Pain, heart-wrenching pain is universal. All the more, I see our mundane existence is actually the state of the world. We are all living a tiny tragedy.

****

Jumping on the Ferris Wheel

December 16 Journal Entry:

Question: Reconciling the sovereignty of God with a tragic event, if God loves me so much, why would He allow an event to cause so much pain to my kids, family, and friends? Scott's students loved him, and he loved them. A huge void was left in their lives, too. Something happens when all the comforters dissipate after a death. They continue with their lives, and you just stand there watching them. They start living again. You don't know where to turn. Like a Ferris wheel. You are trying to jump on while it is going round and round. You see people enjoying the ride. Laughing. Smiling. You *want* to enjoy it, too. It's an enormous task to join them. *How can I get back on this thing?* It won't stop for you. *How do I engineer a plan to jump on?* PTSD throws in another variable. You have weights on your ankles and are tethered to the platform. The weights are the images in your head, and the tether is the panic attacks. So, the carnival continues, and you wait, tethered and chained.

I feel that I have overcome some of those questions. I'm not a Super Christian. I question God often. Perhaps being transparent with the One who sees me clearly has helped. I can sift through these matters of the heart with His gentle, guiding hand. I'm a failure much of the time. I know it. He is patient with my frailties. Having PTSD doesn't mean I can't enjoy life. It just means that my good and bad days look different than the average person's. Someday, I won't have as many intrusive images. Someday, I won't have nightmares three days out of the week. Someday, I will have a day when the incident never enters my mind. Someday.

Has Anyone Seen the Instruction Manual?

I remember the day that I laughed again for the first time. One of those true belly laughs. It was a few months after the accident. It was about three o'clock in the morning. My partner and I were driving back to the station. I don't remember the subject of the conversation, but I recall the laugh. A belly laugh. It was really funny. We laughed for quite a while. Then I felt guilty—guilty that I was happy at that moment, like I didn't deserve to be happy, that I shouldn't be having a good emotion. Then I had an epiphany. I turned to my partner and said, "Thanks, I really needed that." He smiled big and knew exactly what I meant. That was a point in my journey when I knew I was going to make it. I was going to be okay. Someday.

****

This chapter is titled "Has Anyone Seen the Instruction Manual" for a reason. I became a novice at fifty-some years of age. I pretty much had my act together. By fifty you have figured out much of life and are no longer considered the least experienced in the room. Well, that changed. No ducks in a row, just squirrels darting to and fro in traffic.

Some Thoughts

September 22 Journal Entry:

Learning to live with PTSD. How do I battle this without it becoming an excuse—an excuse to shut down, give in, give up, have a pity party, seek sympathy, stay at home, becoming isolated, or fall into anything else that people use PTSD as an excuse for?

Another thought: Can PTSD create symptoms like a cold? Do fatigue, body aches, and malaise come as a package with it? Why do I have good and bad days physically? Maybe it's just my age. Is this forever? Is it brain chemistry?

****

March 19 Journal Entry:

I refer to PTSD as the monster under the bed. But this monster is *real*. That's how I feel about it. It's that mysterious thing that terrifies the bed owner. When I was a child, I was petrified that there was something under my bed that was going to grab my ankle. I would lie there as still as I could, covered up even during sweltering summer days in the second story bedroom with no ventilation. I would have sweat running off my forehead, down my temples onto my pillow. I knew it was there. You are vividly aware of your monster when you feel most vulnerable. You also, or at least I do, feel tormented some days by it even during the day. As a child the monster under the bed grips your soul and heart with fear. It can almost paralyze you like it did to me in my hot bedroom. It's our monster. It's real. It's scary. It's crippling. It's ugly. It's unpredictable. It's sorrow. It's guilt. It's depression. It's shameful. It's unwanted. It's personal. It's my monster. I need to learn how to tame it.

****

Many people will try to hand you an instruction manual. I don't know their motives. One should not delve into the motives behind someone's behavior; that job belongs to the

Has Anyone Seen the Instruction Manual?

Holy Spirit. However, people speak out of ignorance and inexperience. Take it with a grain of salt. The next journal entry explains what I mean.

November 11 Journal Entry:

    I never really spoke openly with anyone in the past because of the fear of judgment. I didn't want Bible verses being tossed at me. I wanted a safe place and a sounding board. I wanted acknowledgment that the struggles were normal and that God could come into that area with healing, not this instant fix or the recipe of "Add Bible verse to problem" and *poof:* problem solved. All better now, so get over it and stop thinking about yourself so much! This doesn't help. A large, broken glass vessel takes time to put all the pieces back together. And what I have learned is that some pieces never fit again. Certain parts of you never become whole until heaven's gate you see.

    This attitude of flinging Bible verses at someone to fix the problem is like throwing tools at a teen and expecting them to repair the brakes on a car. Yes, you gave them a tool, but they have no idea what to do with it. They don't understand the mechanics of it. They *know* something isn't working properly. Asking them to take it apart and put it back together is like rocket science to them. It takes a guiding hand, time, training, and knowledge with a lot of patience. I wish those verse-tossers would wrap their heads around that. And the big question is this: Does the kid even want to learn how to fix the brakes? You can't help someone who doesn't see the problem or is more comfortable with the status quo. So, what do the verse-tossers do? They throw more verses as to why the child needs to fix it. The question should be this: How do I walk alongside this person as they, themselves, discover, with your gentleness, that the problem exists while showing them how to lean into God as they learn His attributes? Letting God do the work. Explaining the tools to them. Showing them how to use the tools. Pushing people to get better, get over it, or get right with God doesn't expose grace. It brings shame and guilt. I'm not saying to withhold the Word of God. I'm saying that it doesn't produce the behavior you want to see. This is a long process and road to walk. It's ugly, tedious, with many battles to be fought. Some won't be won today, tomorrow, or even next year. Don't be a verse-tosser. Be a grace-giver, a walk-besider, a God-attribute-revealer. Explain when they ask. A lot of people like the sound of their own voice too much. Be a listener.

****

Joy. Happiness.

December Journal Entry:

I have been battling depression, lack of sunlight hours, and really no friends except guys at work. They are friends to a point, but there's not the connection I need. I have tried to reach out to some girls but haven't been invited anywhere. Being a loner gets lonely. Have had weird dreams. Have been weepy. Menopause is here, too. *Yay for me.* I cried, sobbed over one of my children's divorce. She (daughter-in-law) was such a part of the family. We have lost her. We have been cut off from her. It hurts.

After the accident, finding happiness was difficult. I desperately want to feel it again. When I did (brief moments), it was a drenching rain amidst a drought. It's fleeting, however. So, I thought about joy instead. Joy is supposed to be what you find from God, and it comes from within, not from outside happenings. Well, let me tell you, joy wasn't found either. Maybe I wasn't doing it right. I yearned to have some good emotion as my circumstances dictated nothing but sorrow and pain. It came back slowly but the sorrow, pain, grief, dreams didn't completely go away. Much of my grief is for my children now—the void I caused them—yes, the guilt is still there. Joy and happiness are still elusive. I've turned into a melancholy.

****

February Journal Entry:

Identity. Let's discuss identity. I went to church alone today. Luke was flying home from work again. We sang many songs from my old church. For the most part I didn't cry or lose my composure. I sat beside a friend. After the service we talked a little more. He complimented me on my voice. I told him that my first husband helped teach me to sing. We spoke a little about our past. He told me his story. He was well on his way to a professional athletic career when he was younger. He identified himself with his athleticism, and when he injured himself, he lost that identity. Then Jesus came. He had no interest in sports or excelling therein. His path changed direction, and he has become very successful in it. He had an interesting story. Most people do, if we would take time to listen, we would gain so much wisdom. I write all that to say this. Identity. This change happens when the monster comes out from beneath the bed.

Before the accident I was the caregiver. The one in charge. The alpha. The shepherd. People would be drawn to me for strength and that caring spirit. I was at the top. (*Maybe this is a reason I was humbled.*) Then, everything changed. I wasn't who

I thought I was. I was a scared little girl. I was weak, vulnerable, and desperate to get away from the people to whom I had a responsibility. I was exhausted by the memories they produced in me. I was trying to create a cushion from my pain. I wasn't strong anymore. In a word, I couldn't *handle* it. I was broken, and my identity was broken along with it.

What's Happening Here?

(Earl)

In this chapter I am going to take a slightly different track. We will still look at some PTSD/CPTSD symptoms; however, I want to focus on the theme of *relationship*. Relationship with God in PTSD/CPTSD, relationship with ourselves, and the non-PTSD/CPTSD relationships toward the ones who suffer from PTSD/CPTSD. I believe this is so important.

Annalise paints the PTSD picture again with bright and vibrant colors. She writes, "Life is messier than a platitude plaque made in China." "PTSD… travels with you. It doesn't stay under the bed. I relive certain aspects from that week every day."

Why is this? The trauma is "downloaded on the brain." The sights, sounds, smells, colors, events are downloaded and stored. That's why things or people or events or scenery can trigger the downloaded movie to play out in our mind's theater again and again and again. Some are memories, but others are flashbacks.

Annalise writes, "You are vividly aware of your monster when you feel most vulnerable."

Annalise asks a great question regarding what to do with the PTSD. She asks, "How do I battle this without it becoming an excuse? An excuse to shut down, give in, give up."

Has Anyone Seen the Instruction Manual?

What do we do? Do we avoid it for a little season? Do we press into it little by little? Do we talk about it? Not talk about it? Go deeper? Embrace some of the anxiety? Get through some of the anxiety? Relax? Fight it? The answer would be *yes*. All of it. There's a time for all of it. There's a place for all of it. There's a need for all of it. There's eventual healing in all of it. This is why PTSDers would do well to be in therapy with a caring and trained professional who can help them identify when the season *is* to do these things. These approaches are all puzzle pieces that eventually make up the picture of healing. I like to say, "There's *a balance* to everything."

What about our relationship with *ourselves* in PTSD/CPTSD? This plays a huge part in healing or setback. More than likely, our relationship with ourselves will fluctuate between bad and good. The goal is to cross the line into *good* and learn to stay there. Annalise describes, "A failed test. This is what it feels like." "I'm not a Super Christian." "By fifty you have figured out much of life and are no longer considered the least experienced in the room. Well, that changed. No ducks in a row, just squirrels darting to and fro in traffic." "Does fatigue, body aches, and malaise come as a package with it (PTSD)?" "And what I have learned is that some pieces never fit again." Here's one: "joy wasn't found either." "This is a long process and road to walk. It's ugly, tedious, with many battles to be fought." "Then I felt guilty." "Trying to make sense of it all." "I'm a failure much of the time." "Having PTSD doesn't mean I can't enjoy life. It just means that my good and bad days look different than the average person's. Someday, I won't have as many intrusive images." "A belly laugh. It was really funny. We laughed for quite a while." "Then I had an epiphany. I turned to my partner and said, 'Thanks, I really needed that.' That was a point in my journey when I knew I was going to make it. I was going to be okay. Someday."

With the above, we can see Annalise's self-talk and how her relationship with herself fluctuated between confusion, upset with herself, humility with reality, changes in her ability, changes in her body, helplessness, loss, guilt/shame, sprouting hope, laughter again, and so on. This is normal and to be expected. With this, if we can learn to accept our brokenness, give ourselves grace in the moments, and not harshly judge ourselves, we can get to a good relationship with ourselves sooner, stay there longer, and begin to grow our roots there. We would treat ourselves like this if we shattered our femur, wouldn't we? We wouldn't beat ourselves up, hate ourselves, and expect ourselves to run a half marathon. Why? Our femur is broken, we're in pain, and we have a cast on. It's common sense. Why is it that we (and unfortunately many others) expect ourselves to "run life's marathon" when we are shattered with PTSD/CPTSD? It's because we can see a cast on a leg, but we can't see emotional brokenness. We don't validate what we cannot see. Nevertheless, the pain of broken emotions is just as painful—or more so—than a broken femur. Let's keep cultivating a good relationship with ourselves by accepting our brokenness, giving ourselves grace in the moment, and not harshly judging ourselves. Also, part of a good relationship with ourselves is not giving ourselves excuses to "run people over" with our words and actions. Let's find ways—healthy ways—to express grief and sorrow and loss and anger that don't include running over those who love us and want to help us.

If you're a loved one or close friend or church member or pastor or coworker of someone with PTSD/CPTSD, then this section is for you. Listen to Annalise's experiences and how she could have been helped on a much deeper level: "People love to tell you how to live. Suggestions fly thick like mosquitos in Alaska." Also, "people speak out of ignorance and inexperience. Take it with a grain of salt." "A lot of people like the sound of their own voice too much. Be a listener." "I never really spoke openly with anyone in the past because of the fear of judgment. I didn't want Bible verses being tossed at me. I wanted a safe place and a sounding board. I wanted acknowledgement that the struggles were normal and that God could come into that area with healing. Not this instant fix or the recipe of 'add Bible verse to problem' and *poof*: problem solved. All better now, now get over it and stop thinking about yourself so much! This doesn't help!" "The question should be this: How do I walk alongside this person… ?" "Something happens when all the comforters dissipate after a death. They continue on with their lives and you just stand there watching them. They start living again. You don't know where to turn." "It's an enormous task to join them."

Now, Annalise is not begrudging people getting back to their lives. She knows they have to work, shop, eat, plan, take the kids to soccer, and have a date night with their spouse. That's all good and okay. She's simply sharing what it's like to see that from the other side of the glass where she can see it but can't touch, experience, or partake of it.

Please take Annalise's advice. Hear her heartbeat regarding helping or hurting by what's said and done. Good, safe relationships are one of the best things to help someone eventually heal from PTSD/CPTSD.

In closing this particular chapter, let's look at the (C) PTSDer's relationship with God. Our relationship is established and made close because of our faith in Jesus. Period. We get a new heart, a new spirit, and God's Spirit at salvation. We get new spiritual DNA. We have new forgiveness, new knowledge, a new relationship. This is the new covenant. With this, we can still carry old thoughts, old patterns, old ways of thinking. These can cause us to *think and feel* something that isn't true—we're failing, God's gotta humble us, or that we've "lost our closeness" and have to "earn our closeness back." I'm sure we'll fluctuate in our relationship with God with some of these thoughts and feelings, too. What we believe about God, however, can propel us more toward healing or bury us in quick-drying cement up to our waist.

What brings closeness, biblically? Blood (Eph. 2:13 NIV). In the Old Testament it was animal blood that could merely cover up sin. In the New Testament it's the blood of Jesus—the perfect sacrifice—that removes sin forever (Heb. 8:12 NIV). The blood of animals was an imperfect shadow of the perfect sacrifice to come. (Devour the book of Hebrews and see!) So, in short, does God "need to teach us a lesson"? Is He needing to "humble us into submission" by throwing traumas at us? Is He really needing to "break us"? With PTSD/CPTSD it sure feels that way at times. But no, He already "killed us" by crucifying us on the cross with Christ when we came to Him by faith however many days or weeks or months or years ago it was. Not only did He do that, but He raised us to newness of life. Not only did He do that, but He seated us in heavenly places in Christ *now*. Is He leading us? Yes. Is He counseling us? Yes. Is He directing us away from certain things and toward other things? Yes. With this, the other mentioned is true, too. Why am I saying this here? It's because how we view God and our relationship to Him can make or break us in our PTSD/CPTSD.

Annalise struggled back and forth with this, too. Take in her words: "Identity. I was at the top. (Maybe this is a reason I was humbled.)" "I question God often. Perhaps being transparent with the One who sees me clearly has helped. I can sift through these matters… with His gentle, guiding hand."

Healing comes with this latter kind of relationship and view of the Father.

Here's something I journaled on December 19, 2022, to process my "closeness" issue and struggle.

Going back to my closeness with God. Is it really about how good I act? How my performance is measured? If I say a swear word in anger privately or swallow it deeply so I don't, and pretend? Is it based on my time spent in prayer—thirty minutes versus ten minutes? Am I closer when I don't feel depressed versus when I do? If I go to four church services per month versus only two? Am I closer because I feel warm and tingly with a certain worship song versus when I feel nothing… but want to feel something? If my closeness is built on this, my closeness to God is like a roller coaster: up and down, twists and turns. This seems like mental and spiritual gymnastics because it is. Some of these things are good and okay things; however, they don't create closeness. *Only blood does that!* Jesus's blood! When I place my faith in Him, and His cross and resurrection become mine on His behalf, and my heart is new because He came in, *this is closeness* to God! Sure, He's counseling my behavior, but my closeness is settled! With a perfect sacrifice, it's gotta be, or it's not a perfect sacrifice. Thank You, Lord Jesus. This is the *truth* that sets me *free*!

You see, we can all get caught up in the religious hamster wheel of always running and running to get close to God, but we're just expending energy trying to get what we already have: closeness with Him.

6
Forward Movement and Containment

At some point I decided to move forward. I do remember that night and situation. It was a tangible moment. I can still see it in my mind. I will hold onto that as I hit rough spots in this journey. I often refer to putting the pieces back together as getting fixed. What if I'm never going to be put back together or fixed? What if I'm just going to be mended? A mended object still has the scars and marks of being broken. Kintsugi is a Japanese art form in which breaks and repairs are treated as part of the object's history. Broken ceramics are carefully mended by mixing resin with gold, silver, or platinum powder. You can still see the repairs. They are beautiful, with the piece sometimes considered more valuable after the repair by the artisans. Kintsugi means "golden joinery." What a beautiful way to look at my life.

New Painting Style

March 23 Journal Entry:

I sold a watercolor today. That's new. People don't buy my art. Mark loved it. I'm saving for a new iPad. This will go into the piggy bank. Stacey wrote this about two of my newest watercolors: "The artwork is stunning. Your work demonstrates a depth of soul and insight that is different than your previous work. Beauty from ashes perhaps?" My paintings have changed. The pedestrian mode is gone. There is something soulful making its way to the surface. Something that doesn't flee from emotions or thought. I am different. I have been rewired, so to speak. I like portions of this rewiring. Now if I can only support my art habit. This new depth of soul has got me thinking. What has changed? What has gotten me to this new place? Scott probably wouldn't have approved of my new style. Bold and strange colors, scantily clad models or some other creative mood I have been in. Raw and dark. Expressive and conversational. I would like to think that I see things a bit differently. My dad just had cataract surgery. He stated that the old lens he was looking through distorted the true colors. After surgery the colors are brighter and not at all what he has been looking at for these last several years. He said that it's amazing. I feel sort of the same way in some areas of life. Purpose. Time spent well. Clutter. Material possessions. Family. Grace. I put each one in its own sentence because I wanted to park on each one as a complete statement. It is its own subject and predicate. Our very short life. Our life is but a vapor according to the Bible. How true. I refuse to pursue things any longer. I refuse to procrastinate when it comes to spending time with family. I refuse to stay angry. I refuse to think of myself as anything but blessed. I live with the struggle of regrets. I am not going to waste my love. I am walking through anxiety without pity or a defeated attitude.

****

Some additional thoughts:

Forward Movement and Containment

I called this chapter "Forward Movement and Containment." Forward means that my focus is ahead. I recall a day very clearly in my mind. I went to the cemetery. We'd decided to purchase a plot so we would have some place to go to grieve, to have his name in stone. Even though he was lost to the water, we wanted a tangible place to gather. I was having a conversation with God while standing at his headstone. Tears streamed down my cheeks. I can't remember what the day was about. I don't remember why I came to the grave, even. Maybe to talk to Scott. I just know it was after I decided that I needed to live and live well. I am crying as I'm writing this—tears for grace and from deep sorrow. I begged God to help me. I wanted comfort and protection. I wanted to move forward. I believe I asked for Him to take the pain away, the images, too. A strong wind came up and literally dried my tears. In the wind I could sense His presence and comfort. He was drying my tears and pushing me onward. I raised my head, faced into the wind, and let the tears evaporate. I stood there, face toward the sky, wind flowing through my hair. I walked to my car, drove off, and when I looked in the rearview mirror to see the headstone, I was reminded of why the mirror is small and the windshield is big. I don't like to get all mushy like this, but it was a forward moment for me.

Another Book

Journal Entry:

Signed papers today. My house has sold. That book is closed. I guess I have had that perspective about many things these past few years. It's not another chapter in my life; it's a whole new book. College, another book. New job, another book. Houses, another book. Grandmotherhood, another book. New husband, another book. When I look at it in that light, it gives a sense of newness. The old book has been written, finished, and placed on a shelf. Occasionally I reach for it, cradle it in my hands, and read from its pages. I did that today. I cried on the way to the signing. I called Luke, and we talked about it a bit. When I got there, I was all smiles and had no emotion. Emotion Thief, anyone? Either way, I'm glad this new family will fill my house with love, children, and laughter. Closing the book again and placing it on that shelf.

****

During this forward motion I have had to ask myself the hard question. Excuses?

January Journal Entry:

Learning to live with PTSD. How do I battle this without it becoming an excuse? Excuse to shut down, give in, give up, pity myself, and seek sympathy. Become isolated because of the pain? Doing the easy thing? The easy thing makes a path for the excuses. I cannot let myself become a victim of my own mind. Pain is not going to be an excuse for me to hide away.

****

Part of moving forward is letting go of my plans.

January Journal Entry:

Sick today. Common cold. Death has been on my mind lately. So many people I love are experiencing the loss of someone. Fathers, grandpas, close friends (young and old), even pets. Death is part of being alive. Everything dies. Sometimes it happens before we think it should. When my expectations are smashed, it adds another dimension to the pain. When death is the result of a long struggle with an illness, it's not a surprise, which is not to say that the pain is any less. When that doctor gives the diagnosis and a time frame you can put things in order. People are called. Families gather. They say the goodbyes and hold the hands. But when a life ends without a heads-up, it takes on a different face. I don't know which I prefer. Each is terrible. Either you grieve for months or years before the death or it hits you like a hammer in the stomach. I choose neither. In my world, nobody dies. We all wait for our Lord's return. When I superimpose my vision of this world on top of God's plan, I have created an idolatrous world. I cannot see what His plan is. I do not know why He allows this pain. To take away all this would mean that I'm running the show. I have to let go of my plans and vision for my life. This is not easy. My heart desperately knows how much I need God and His love and strength. I need His comfort. Perhaps the anxiety is the unresolved within me. The expectations versus reality. God is slowly and gently bringing those exposing thoughts to the mediation table. Two enemies of state. Will it take years? Decades? Never? All I know is that He will sit at the table for as long as I need.

****

Understand the loss of expectations.

April Journal Entry:

Are shattered dreams and expectations a loss? Do people grieve the loss? In my opinion, yes. When one of my children was diagnosed with a chronic disease, I went through a grieving period. I mourned. I cried a lot. I mourned the loss of a normal, healthy childhood. Everything that they will face. It was a great, continuing loss. I am realizing that with my traumatic event came loss on a number of fronts. The obvious was the death of my husband, but there were other losses that I didn't even recognize yet. How could I know that friendships change? The great void of identity? How about the loss of confidence in your ability to function? The future. The dreams of retirement. Family vacations. Projects that will never be done. Seeing that wrench left on the garage floor, right where he placed it during an unfinished project. He was fixing my car. It didn't get done. When I was cleaning out my house, a friend found the tote where I kept my wedding dress. I was inspecting every box to see if I needed to throw it out. She stopped me. "You don't want to look in there." She then told me why. I broke down, and a deluge of memories of our wedding day buried me. I sat on the dirty steps and sobbed a gut-wrenching sob. Another crushing blow. *No more wedding anniversaries.* And the big ones are family. That empty chair during holidays. The weddings not attended. The expectations of being grandparents. Not only did we lose him, we lost all that the future holds. I mourned the expectations. And that grief seems to have lasted longer. Every milestone in my children's lives is a reminder of that unfulfilled expectation. It's like baking. I thought I was supposed to be baking banana bread. I felt as if it was an episode of *Chopped*.

Forward Movement and Containment

The basket of ingredients was not what I imagined. Apparently, I'm not baking banana bread. I'm baking something entirely different. In this moment I muster the strength to be thankful and praise Him for the new ingredients. I will do this today, but tomorrow I will be angry and frustrated with the new recipe.

****

Additional thoughts:

Unrealized expectations are a lot like baking. Follow the recipe and your banana bread will be foolproof. We like recipes. Measure this, blend that, add a smidgin of bam, bake at such and such for just so long, and you get the delicious outcome for all to enjoy. But what if the ingredients were taken away and you still wanted to bake the same recipe? What then? Frustration and a nasty-tasting concoction. Or find a different recipe that includes that zucchini, avocado, and sardine (*yuck*!) you were handed. You can still have a yummy dish; it just takes flexibility to change your expectations of the cuisine. I have learned to expect very little to go the way I want it to. We've all been slapped in the face too many times to think otherwise. Water off a duck's back. Let it roll. Be flexible. God changes the ingredients; turn the page of the cookbook.

I used the word *containment* in the title of this chapter. My dictionary app gives a couple definitions:

1. An act of policy of restricting the territorial growth or ideological influence of another, especially a hostile nation.
2. An act of policy of limiting the expansion or spread of a natural disaster, contagion, or other dangerous thing.

3. In a nuclear power plant, an enclosure completely surrounding a nuclear reactor, designed to prevent the release of radioactive material in the event of an accident.

I would liken my panic and anxiety to the nuclear power plant. I would have a meltdown. A number of years after the incident, my counselor referred to containment. He stated that I am in containment mode. I am not having the meltdowns that I once had. I am not having as much panic, and the need for medication during the day has diminished greatly. I am able to work. I am getting better? Am I fixed? Not by a long shot. I'm just containing the disaster better.

Building the Walls of Containment

May Journal Entry:

Containment. Interesting thought. Earl used that word today. As time goes by, grief and PTSD are still there; it's just contained. I know how tall and thick to build those containment barriers. I know what may trigger the panic. I know what starts to feel familiar. I take the necessary steps to ensure the dam won't break and all that ugliness comes pouring out. It's the unknown, unfamiliar, uncharted, and surprises that leave me defenseless. Like that morning I knew someone had been in my car. I was blindsided, unprepared for that panic assault. No time to put barriers up. Totally unprotected. I have experienced a great amount of healing, don't get me wrong. What I'm trying to convey is that the wound is always there and tender. Containment is what helps me combat the times when it gets bumped, scraped, or reopened. Containment can be with God or without Him. Without Him will work in the short term but is exhausting. With Him, peace and comfort can be readily available. (Both will be hard, but with Him there's the long-term benefit of healing that comes from Him.) That acknowledgment that there is a wound. How many times have I tried to be tough, pretending that I have no wound? I should take my own advice and work toward God-containment. Easy to write. Not as easy in the moment of wall building. When panic arrives, it takes my rationale and boots it out the door. I'm glad God is forward facing. There are more blessings ahead. Am I poised to accept them?

****

Something like Tourette's?

May Journal Entry:

Saw Earl today. Good session. I didn't totally understand what Earl was talking about when he said "containment mode." We talked about it again today. Now I understand an analogy of containment better. I likened it to someone with Tourette's. Dear friends of mine have a child with Tourette's. We were talking the other day about how difficult it can be for their daughter to hold in her tics at school. She works hard at it. Then, when she gets home it's bad. She will have long periods of the tics and it's exhausting for her. It struck a chord with me. I feel as if I'm building containment walls or containers. (Duh, Annalise). I'm holding in my little grains of anxiety, memories, smells, tastes, and fears. Unfortunately, containment only goes so far. There's a crack. There's a breach. There has to be a relief valve on that boiler. I can only hold it in so long before there will be an episode. Sometimes I can control the breach. It takes so much emotional energy to keep composure. Maybe like tics. You ask, "Isn't this life? Doesn't everyone break?" Well, I can honestly say that I had few, and they were nothing like what I experience now. The straws on the camel are made of lead, and the camel's back has been weakened by circumstances that I didn't choose. This is not a pity-grabbing exploitation. This is what I experience. This is my normal. I would be the first one to change it if I could. After four years, I thought that I would be "better." No, I'm just maintaining containment. I have noticed that the containment walls have gotten thicker and have held more. God's grace and mercy sometimes scoop out the rubbish within the walls. Sometimes, He allows the walls to crack and spill. I have no answer to why. I could rattle on about some spiritual enlightenment on this matter, but it would be a lie.

****

Future, Past, Present.

June Journal Entry:

Have been working a lot this week to put the new house together. Spent the better part of the day sorting, searching, cleaning, and rummaging through boxes. I found my antique serving dishes! Finally, my kitchen and dining table are starting to reflect me. My stuff, my dishes. It's been over two years since I have touched this stuff. I find it strange that we identify ourselves with material objects. Cars, trucks, artwork, Gramma's jewelry, land, even serving bowls are woven into our being. For a long time I felt as if I had no tangible thing to anchor me. They were all in boxes. Limbo. I was using someone else's dishes.

Forward Movement and Containment

I feel more myself than I have in a long time. I'm no longer living in another woman's home. Even though Luke's wife passed many years ago, her style and decor choices were still there. It really wasn't pleasant. Lately, I've been pondering the adage to "roll like water off a duck's back." As my house went to a different family, I am learning to accept change. I never expected my life to be turned upside down. Such an unexpected ride. I think of the carnival ride that I was never allowed to go on. It was called Salt and Pepper Shakers. You start out just going round and round in a bullet-shaped cage mounted to a large steel beam. Two opposing cages going high, then low. It goes faster, and then the unexpected happens: the cages start to spin. Those little ten year olds start to scream. Next thing you know, there's puke. Thanks, Mom and Dad. You were right. No one expected the spin. I've really had a boring life, but a good life. Uneventful. Same work schedule, same church times, same meals, same vacations, same struggles, irritations, marital squabbles, same, same, same. Then came that moment when the cage starts to spin. Strange, I knew it the second after he was gone. My mind raced—raced to everything I would have to do. It seemed as though in those eternal moments while screaming, "Noooooooo," I had the weight of this enormous mental picture of the future. I had been on many cardiac arrests and other deaths to know what had to be done. It was daunting. The details of death were looming. If inflexibility was in my character, God was going to force it out of me. Priorities became crystal clear. I wish I could change some of the events that occurred after the accident. I wish my kids and I would have held each other more. I wish we could have snuggled on the couch instead of retreating to separate rooms to grieve. Everyone has regrets in times like this.

****

Living in the Vapor

May Journal Entry:

    Just finished my work week. Only thirty-one hours. People have asked why I don't apply for the full-time position. I talked with Luke about it. We both agreed that it probably wouldn't be the best for us. With his work taking him away many days of the week, we felt it would not be good for us as a couple to see each other even less than what we do. Life is more than work, church activities, sewing, vacations, or health insurance. It's a balance. I am trying to balance what is important and what is necessary. Luke and I decided that together.

    My family is more important than the money. I'm very blessed to have that option. I know some women aren't. If I wouldn't have met Luke, I would have had to apply for the full-time slot and worked my tail off to save my house. Actually, there was no saving my house. I could not have kept it even if my children were helping to pay the mortgage and expenses. I was accepting the future of a tiny efficiency apartment in the city. I choose to see the goodness in this. It hasn't been an easy road. I'm sure my children think I remarried too soon. Interestingly enough, his children felt the same way. The people who didn't think so were the older people: our parents, older pastors, older friends who were widowed. These people understand the brevity of life.

    I need to think about that for a moment. How did I get here so quickly? Late fifties. How did my grandparents pass so soon? Or my friends? This life is short. The days seem long whilst the decades whiz past me. Our life is truly a vapor. So, how do I live in the vapor? How does someone come out on the other side of a traumatic event in a healthy manner? If I have learned anything, it is the question, "What's important?" What *is* important?

God, of course, and people. Your job would be given to someone else before you finish a load of laundry. Your things will be parted out or thrown out before the grave has new grass. Houses will fall in, becoming dilapidated. Cars, motorcycles, and big-people toys will rust. Church programs will go on without you. The important stuff isn't stuff, as the adage goes. Petty family squabbles are a waste of time. The things that I thought I had to fight about and make my point on are meaningless. Perhaps this is why Luke and I don't bicker. We are so thankful for each other, so we treat each other as a gift from God. When I live in the vapor, I am acutely aware of the brevity of life and want my life to reflect that. What does thankfulness do for me? It changes my pattern of thinking. My glass is neither half empty or half full. It's always *being* filled. It isn't always easy. Some days I can only see the empty portion of the glass. It takes effort to see past the storm clouds. Many times I don't see the sun. I literally cry out to God with my lament. Occasionally He will part the clouds so I can see a glimmer. Sometimes, many times, He doesn't. I'm not going to pretend that the days of depression go away that quickly. Sometimes I just go to bed and look forward to a different tomorrow. Sometimes I am angry (seething rage is actually a better word for what I feel). However, I do not label myself. I'm not a widow, or a victim of circumstance, a failure, or a single mom, at least not today. My mind is in a fluid state. This has made me feel like a helpless little girl and also an empowered, independent woman. If anything, I'm a survivor. With survivor's guilt. Living in the vapor.

****

Final thought:

Kintsugi. That pottery repair thingy with gold or platinum. I would like to think of myself as a piece of kintsugi pottery. God allowed something to shatter me. I would like to believe that the holes are filled with precious metal. I have to remind myself that I am His and the event that shattered my life is being filled. I was reminded again last week that my life is going in a different direction than it was a number of years ago. I have a different calling as a wife, mother, stepmother, and grandmother. My roles are different. I have a different sphere of influence now. Even though I'm broken, really broken some days, I am here for a reason. God has revealed some of His plan as to the *"Why?"* I'm not happy that PTSD is part of that package. If it were me, I would have done it differently. However, I would still be ignorant. I would still be too proud to admit I don't have all the answers. Before all this, I didn't know I was broken. After, as painful as it continues to be, I realize how messed up I am. I have more patience and compassion; I'm less judgmental. The break creates the beauty of kintsugi. Maybe that's what I needed to be a beautiful soul.

What's Happening Here?

(Earl)

The progression of these chapters by Annalise couldn't have been more perfect. This last chapter led right to the idea of post-traumatic growth, as it has been called. This is the idea that PTSD/CPTSD is real and horrible; with this, it doesn't have to stop there. It can be like kintsugi, where beauty and strength

Forward Movement and Containment

can reside in the broken places. This by no means invalidates the reality and horror of PTSD/CPTSD; it just adds that life doesn't have to be over either. It lends the element of hope and balance.

Let's review the messages of hope and post-traumatic growth that Annalise artistically laid out for us in this chapter. She writes, "At some point I decided to move forward." Yes, moving forward is a decision just like staying stuck is a decision. This is a privileged decision we PTSDers get to make. Now, is it easy? No. Will we vacillate in this decision? Yes, in the beginning. Does making the decision to move forward communicate that the trauma wasn't really that big of a deal? No. The trauma was a huge deal. Does it mean one is in denial? No. It's healthy to want to get our life back. Is suggesting to move forward invalidating the hurt and grief and hit of the trauma(s)? One hundred times, no. It's communicating that the trauma happened, it hurt, it was devastating, it ran over us ten thousand times, and we were "knocked out." Because of this, we want to have the privilege of getting our lives back again. Hopefully, this is what it communicates to those warriors with PTSD/CPTSD. This is how Annalise and I mean it, anyway.

She said, "I will hold on to that as I hit rough spots in this journey." Yes, there will be rough spots. Not *if* but *when*. When the turbulence is felt, going back to the desire and the privilege and the beauty of getting our life back is something to hold on to. This helpful commitment can make desire a reality in time. What's our *beauty*? Our spouse? Children? Both? Our job? A BFF? Our pet? Hiking in the woods on a crisp fall day? The mountains? Water? A good book by the fireplace? The deer that makes their way into our yard at dusk? That perfect cup of coffee? More than likely, our *beauty* is a combination of half a dozen things. During those turbulent times, going back to the beauty in our lives can be an anchor during times of anger, addiction, temptations, anxiety, withdrawing, arguing, or whatever it is. We can begin to replace the chaos with the beauty of more silence and calm as we engage in the *beauty* of our lives. In therapy, this is one aspect of mindfulness: finding meaning in the present moment.

Analise comments, "A mended object still has the scars and marks of being broken." Yes. As in the art work kintsugi, beauty like integrity, understanding, patience, depth, wisdom, compassion, and strength can show through the cracks and broken pieces of PTSD/CPTSD in our lives. Do those cracks and broken pieces still hurt at times? You bet! With it, the beauty and strength showing through these cracks and broken pieces as we get our lives back will be evident, too. As the saying goes: "We can get bitter, or we can get better." Now, we will get bitter for a season. I'm going to look at this as it's our way of validating the trauma(s), grieving the trauma(s), being angry at the unfairness of the trauma(s). Staying in this season will eventually destroy us, though. There comes another season that is a good season to transition into as well. It's the season of *better*, of getting on the path of getting our life back. This is what Annalise is talking about.

Here's another example of the above: "Stacey wrote this about two of my newest paintings: 'The artwork is stunning. Your work demonstrates a depth of soul and insight that is different than your previous paintings. Beauty from ashes perhaps?'" Again, Kintsugi. God doesn't cause all the traumas we may face; however, He doesn't let it go to waste. He uses it and us.

Hear Annalise's joy: "I sold a watercolor today. That's new. People don't buy my art. I'm saving for a new iPad. This will go into my piggy bank." This is an awesome analogy of Annalise's post-traumatic growth (though this was an actual event). I see it as a symbol:

(a) Annalise did something new—she sold a watercolor painting. This was a new step in her journey.
(b) She was saving her money for an iPad. The reward for selling something was going toward something else.

The reward of us getting our life back "goes toward" a healthier life, better mental health, closer relationships, possibly addiction-free living, more in-depth social life, resuming loved hobbies that have been set aside, and more. To gain something, sometimes we have to let something else go. Again, this is *not* to invalidate and say, "Just get the heck over it, man!" No way!

When we get to the place where we desire to get some of our life back, that's when our grip of the past begins to loosen so we can "use that hand" to grab ahold of something better, more precious. Look at Annalise's "new grip": "I refuse to pursue things any longer. I refuse to procrastinate when it comes to spending time with family. I refuse to stay angry. I refuse to think of myself as anything but blessed. I live with the struggle of regrets. I am not going to waste my love. I am working through anxiety without pity and a defeated attitude."

Annalise is ready! She knows the reality of pain, and rightly so. She knows the value (and heartache) of grief, and she will continue, which is good and needed. She has seen the "time thief" that has placed cement shoes on her feet and caused her to walk slowly in life, which is normal. Now, she also wants to embrace the "other normal" and love, spend quality time, see the good too, and navigate through the triggers and emotions rather than be buried by them. Again, she will continue to grieve on and off. This is good, healthy, and normal. When our thoughts, emotions, and body tell us, "Hey, we need out, and we need some attention here." Yes, it's right and good to give them our attention and grieve and mourn. John Eldredge, author of *Wild at Heart*, says that a wound not grieved is a wound that won't heal. We must *go there*.

Annalise has *gone there* and will *go there*. Listen: "In this moment I muster the strength to be thankful and praise Him for the new ingredients. I will do this today, but tomorrow I will be angry and frustrated with the new recipe." "I have learned to expect very little to go the way I want it to." "How many times have I tried to be tough, pretending that I have no wound?" "I'm holding in my little grains of anxiety, memories, smells, tastes, and fears. Unfortunately, containment only goes so far. There's a crack. There's a breach. There has to be a relief valve on that boiler. I can only hold it in so long before there will be an episode."

She has *gone there*. She just wants to *go to the other (good and beautiful) places, too*. Annalise isn't ignoring the past; she's just seeing the future bigger. She says, "I… drove off, and when I looked in the rearview mirror to see the headstone, I was reminded of why the mirror is small and the windshield is big." Again, post-traumatic growth.

For believers in Jesus Christ, here's the blessing of partnership with Him: we don't have to do *any* of this alone. He is a good counselor, friend, master rebuilder. Annalise writes, "A strong wind came up and literally dried my tears." Annalise experienced a symbol of Jesus being that good counselor, friend, master rebuilder. God can use symbols in our lives. For my wife it has been sun rays coming through during hard times. Annalise's symbol wasn't God saying that tears aren't good. Her symbol was that God sees the tears, so go ahead and cry, and He will help wipe them away, as well.

Annalise writes, "Perhaps the anxiety is unresolved within me." This is key. As humans we tend to do one of two things—we explode, or we stuff/hide. Both are unhealthy extremes. What's in the middle? The middle is to *go to* those uncomfortable, dark, scary, unwanted places from time to time when needed to eventually *resolve* it. Notice I didn't say *end it* but *resolve it*. The trauma won't end with our religious or psychological formulas. *Do A and you'll get B!* But there are things that have been proven that we can put in place so we can eventually resolve (not forget but live with) it. That's what post-traumatic growth is *eventually*. *Eventually* healing more, *eventually* living more, *eventually* looking through the windshield more and the rearview mirror less, *eventually* seeing the trauma moving to the side rather than being in the center, *eventually* getting more and more of our lives back again. This is a gradual journey, not a quick rocket ride. To me, this is freeing. The pressure to "be fixed" is off.

Let's look at other of Annalise's writings that show her path of post-traumatic growth: "It's not another chapter in my life, it's a whole new book. University, another book. New job, another book. Houses, another book. Grandmotherhood, another book. New husband, another book. When I look at it in that light, it gives a sense of newness. The old book has been written, finished, and placed on a shelf. Occasionally I reach for it, cradle it in my hands, and read from its pages. Closing the book again and placing it on that shelf."

Also, "Learning to live with PTSD" and "How do I battle this without it becoming an excuse? An excuse? Excuse to shut down, give in, give up, pity myself, and seek sympathy. Become isolated because of the pain? Doing the easy thing? The easy thing makes a path for the excuse. I cannot let myself become a victim of my own mind. Pain is not going to be an excuse for me to hide away."

Again, "Part of moving forward is letting go of my plans." Let's camp here for a moment. Pain hurts! Life can stink terribly at times! Trauma is, well, traumatic! These are rightfully uncomfortable! Valid! Worthy of grief and mourning! Along with this, drugs, alcohol, rage, sexual promiscuity, withdrawing for long periods of time, cheating on your spouse to "kill the pain," ignoring the kids, and getting overweight and unhealthy are on the path to excuses, to nothingness, to hiding. This is not invalidation. This is to simply say that your life is *way more* than these things to your family, friends, yourself possibly, and to God. You matter—terrified you, hurt you, self-hated you. You matter.

Here are other excerpts from Annalise's journal: "I have experienced a great amount of healing, don't get me wrong. What I'm trying to convey is that the wound is always there and tender." "All I know is that He" (God) "will sit at the table for as long as I need." "I am learning to accept change." "Life is more than work, church activities, art, vacations, or health insurance. It's a balance. I am trying to balance what is important and what is necessary." "I'm very blessed to have that option." "I choose to see the goodness in this." "This life is short." "If I have learned anything, it is the question, 'What's important?'" "We are so thankful for each other, so we treat each other as a gift from God." "What does thankfulness do for me? It changes my pattern of thinking." "If anything, I am a survivor. With survivor's guilt. Living in the vapor." "My roles are different. I have a different sphere of influence now. Even though I'm broken, really broken some days, I am here for a reason." "I have more patience and compassion; I'm less judgmental. The break creates the beauty of kintsugi."

Three words to all this: *wow, wow,* and *wow.* This is available to all of us PTSDers. Yes, at different speeds, in some different ways. With this, it's available. Annalise found it. I found it. You can find it.

This is *not* to say *we have to be healed in order to be somebody, be right, or be worth something!* Absolutely not! We are those things *now*, broken and unhealed. It's just that we were meant for more. We were meant for restoration, for healing, for kintsugi to let others see the beauty in our brokenness that was mended together, with cracks visible but gold in their place.

Thank you, Annalise, for your raw courage through your transparency and vulnerability. You *went back there* so you could help others *go back there* to see God create the "art of kintsugi" in their lives through embracing the difficult path and seeing the grace of Jesus Christ "fill the cracks with pure gold."

In the following few chapters, I (Earl) will look at some practical, proven psychological steps we PTSDers can embark on that can eventually bring some of the healing we need.

Thank you.

7
Where to Begin?

Where do we even begin with identifying the building blocks of PTSD/CPTSD and eventually our recovery? If I'm 100 percent honest, I'm not 100 percent sure. Formulas aren't my strong point. People are different. However, I have a pretty good idea.

First, unfortunately, trauma is a part of life. Life is full of good and bad things that happen to us. We laugh, joke, enjoy, and play. We also hurt, grieve, cry, and, in some cases, develop PTSD/CPTSD. Like a good Clint Eastwood movie, life is *The Good, The Bad, and The Ugly*. No way around this. For some, the good, bad, or ugly is more intense, more severe, and more often than for others. It depends on what has happened to us. It's all real, and the effects are real in each of our lives.

Second, our brain is like the highest-tech computer. It records, stores, plays back, rehearses, and "freezes" with things that have happened. Personally, I believe part of this is because the brain's job is to protect us. It tells us, "Hey, remember what happened! Tread lightly! Be careful! That destroyed you! That hurt! Don't do that again! Be afraid!" Hence, we listen to the advice. In some cases, rightly so. Where it gets off balance is when we listen too much to our brain's warnings and advice—especially in cases when it may not be warranted. This causes mental, emotional, physical, and spiritual paralysis. We freeze, get stuck, can't move, or we get the heck out of dodge! Or we fight like a wolverine with nothing to lose. PTSDers can fight, flight, or freeze when it may not be warranted.

Third, there are triggers that cause our fears to pop up. People a lot smarter than I am who have studied the brain say that the brain doesn't distinguish between real threat and perceived threat. It sees it all as a *threat*. For example, let's say that someone was jumped, beaten up, and robbed by four men. That's an assault. Let's say that years later this same person is taking a leisurely walk on a nice summer night. They see four men up ahead walking toward them. The brain is going to trigger this person, yelling, "Warning!" in their head and soul. However, when these four men approach, they turn out to be four elderly men—grandpas—who are out for a walk enjoying each other's company. No threat in the least. However, the brain of the trauma victim looked at this as a definite threat. This is the "amygdala hijack" discussed in chapter 3. We get the idea.

Fourth, triggers cause the fight, flight, or freeze response with a behavior that follows. I remember years ago when I was in a seminar. One of the individuals made a comment, an innocent comment, that triggered me and caused the fight, flight, or freeze response. Right then and there, my mind took me back to a traumatic incident I experienced a few years prior. Rationally I knew I wasn't back in that situation; however, every emotional fiber in my being felt like I was back in that trauma. I wanted to bolt out of that seminar. I wanted to run. I chose to sit there (didn't really have a choice), feel the fear, navigate through it, calm myself with some self-talk, and realize my amygdala was trying to hijack my logical brain. I knew that within about twenty minutes my brain would cool down. The fear at that

Where to Begin?

time didn't fully go away because I was newly applying my coping skills; however, it subsided a little.

Behaviors follow. What are some behaviors that follow our triggers at times? Addiction? Anger that leads to fights/arguing? Withdrawing? Passivity? Spending money we don't have? Believing our inner critic? Affairs? Porn? Letting ourselves be taken advantage of? How we deal with our triggers will determine what positive or negative behaviors we will choose to engage in. This is not a reprimand; it's just reality.

Fifth, our behaviors cause consequences, good or bad. Anger is normal with PTSD. With this, harsh, heavy, cutting, consistent berating and fighting with our spouse can severely fracture a relationship or end in divorce. If these uncontrolled emotional outbursts are directed toward our children, we can damage our relationship and cause undue fear and trauma with them. If it's toward coworkers, it can cause us to get fired. On and on we can go. We may fear ending up all alone, but that's what can happen in cases like this.

Sixth, consequences cripple us or care for us. If we choose to self-medicate with alcohol, drugs, porn, affairs, or whatever, the consequences cripple us and limit where we can go in life in many ways. Unhealthy expressions of anger (not all expressions are unhealthy) can cause others to bolt, and we end up isolated and with a lot of emotional and physical discomfort. If we admit our struggle(s), or we are courageous enough to be vulnerable and get the help we need, we can have a more positive outcome. Our consequences from our choices can shape us and our lives toward the negative or toward the positive. In turn, we can become either a mentor to others or a tormentor to others. We are a helper or a hinderer. We can be a shattered vessel that shatters others, or we can be kintsugi pottery that shows gold in the broken places.

Again, these ideas aren't meant to be a reprimand at all. They are meant to be a help as we navigate through a very real part of our lives: the traumatic experiences that may forever shape our lives and how we respond to them.

Try to identify the following areas:

What are the traumatic experiences in your life that have developed your PTSD/CPTSD?

_____
_____
_____
_____
_____
_____
_____
_____
_____
_____
_____
_____

What are some of the events that your brain has recorded, stored, plays back, gets stuck on?

_____
_____

Where to Begin?

What are the triggers that cause your fear or anger or other symptoms to pop up?

Are you in fight, flight, or freeze mode, or are you frozen in a combination of these? What does the fight, flight, or freeze look like to you?

_____
_____
_____
_____
_____
_____
_____
_____
_____

What behaviors tend to follow a triggering experience?

_____
_____
_____
_____
_____
_____
_____
_____

Where to Begin?

Can you identify the consequences to your behaviors when you've been triggered? Are these consequences crippling you or caring for you?

How are consequences from your choices shaping you and your life?

Is this the kind of life you want to live? If not, what does the kind of life you want to live really look like?

How do you get to the kind of life you want to be living and to the kind of person you want to be? I believe the next chapters can help us PTSDers/CPTSDers begin to answer this question and will give us the practical tools to see this having an effect in our lives.

8

Practical Helps to Get the Kind of Life We Want: Understanding Our Brain and How It Works

There are a variety of things that can help us in our recovery of PTSD/CPTSD. I want to consider two things: the physiology of the brain and our thinking. The first is how the brain works in fear or stress, and the second is referred to as cognitive behavioral therapy (or CBT) and cognitive processing therapy (CPT). Now, it has been determined that CBT is not the best modality when it comes to PTSD/CPTSD. In a nutshell, CBT is *thinking about what we're thinking about.* In other words, it's exploring our ways of thinking to see if they (our thoughts) are harmful or helpful to our overall mental health. With this, if CBT can help 25 to 30 percent, then I want that 25 to 30 percent. It has helped me to a fair degree in my navigation through CPTSD. So, let's use the 25 to 30 percent that CBT can bring. CPT is used more for trauma. CPT, in short, helps us identify our triggers more and to work through our distress. (We will look at CBT and CPT in another chapter. To get back to the thinking part of the brain, there needs to be some "cool down" that will be helpful to review first.)

Regarding the physiology of the brain. In Daniel Goleman's book *Emotional Intelligence,* regarding emotional hijacking, he writes, "But circuits from the limbic brain to the prefrontal lobes mean that the signals of strong emotion—anxiety, anger, and the like—can create neural static, sabotaging the ability of the prefrontal lobe to maintain working memory. That is why when we are emotionally upset we say we 'just can't think straight'—and why continual emotional distress can create deficits… crippling the capacity to learn" (page 27).

In his seminar, Daniel Goleman explains the amygdala (a part of our brain function) as "the alarm center" of our brain. It asks, "Am I safe?" He says, "It's the brain's radar for threat." He continues to say that the amygdala says, "I'd rather be safe than sorry!" The amygdala hijack is in three stages, per Daniel Goleman. One, there's a sudden negative emotional reaction. This comes from what we experience—a situation. Two, it creates a very strong emotional reaction—really angry, really anxious, or really fearful. Three, we do something we really regret afterward, whether it's something we do or say.

Amygdala hijack will occur when we feel strong emotions take over the thinking part of our brain. These emotions can be fear, anxiety and anger. This can trigger the fight/flight/freeze/fawn response.

This gives us a pretty good working definition of amygdala hijack.

Here is a word picture of the amygdala hijack that I've heard in part. Some of it is original to me. Picture the brain as an airplane. The prefrontal cortex is the pilot. It navigates and flies the plane, our brain. It's capable and reliable. Now, way back in the plane is a passenger. Their name is "Amygdala." Amygdala is there to warn of any danger. Sometimes, though, the "danger"

Understanding Our Brain and How It Works

that this passenger reports is just *perceived danger*. So, imagine the plane has taken off. You're flying the friendly skies. All of a sudden, Amygdala sees strong lightning in the not-too-far distance. Fear and anxiety pumps through Amygdala's veins, and they get out of their seat, rush down the aisle, and kick open the cockpit door. Amygdala apprehends the pilot (the prefrontal cortex, the logical thinking part of the brain) and ties them up. Amygdala takes over the pilot's job but doesn't do a good job because it's not amygdala's function. So, the ride is choppy, and the plane is losing altitude because of the unskilled Amygdala. Amygdala has hijacked the plane, taking it way off its route. It's a choppy and dangerous flight now, so buckle up and hold on tight! This is the physiology of the brain during fear, stress, anxiety, and anger that I remember hearing about many years ago.

Since 1961, we've had air marshals who accompany flights to ensure the safety of the flight and passengers. I refer to the air marshal as stress-relieving exercises that are proven psychological treatments that significantly help. Now, these exercises may not be a cure-all. With this, they can offer significant help in "cooling off the troubled brain."

Let's put it this way: as we engage in some of these psychological and stress relieving exercises, it's the air marshal who walks down the aisle, apprehends the amygdala, puts the amygdala back in the plane as a passenger, unties the real pilot, refreshes him, and puts the pilot back in the pilot's seat to fly the plane again. The plane gains altitude, gets back on route, smooths out, and then the seatbelt sign turns off at last. We're back to "flying the friendly skies."

When the brain sees or perceives threat, it affects our autonomic nervous system (ANS). According to Wayne Weiten, Dana S. Dunn, and Elizabeth Yost Hammer in their book *Psychology Applied to Modern Life, Adjustment in the 21st Century, Tenth Edition,* the autonomic nervous system is subdivided into the *sympathetic division* and the *parasympathetic division,* or what's referred to as the *sympathetic* and *parasympathetic.* The sympathetic state puts us in what has been called the fight/flight/freeze mode. (Recently, I heard another "f" they are adding called "fawning," which means to please and appease the perpetrator.) This state prepares our body to fight back, get the heck out of dodge, or freeze. The parasympathetic state is when we are calm and relaxed. Both states affect our body's functioning. We cannot be in both states at the same time. Our goal when things are good but the brain is telling us things are not good is to move to the parasympathetic state. This comes by the thoughts and stress-relieving exercises we will explore.

Can you identify how you feel and what happens to you specifically when your amygdala hijack happens?

_____
_____
_____
_____
_____
_____
_____
_____
_____
_____

The next chapter will focus on these proven psychological and stress-relieving exercises to give our brain the cooling down and relief we need so that we can re-engage the thinking part of our brain.

9

Practical Helps to Get the Kind of Life We Want: Proven Stress-Relieving Exercises

The following are proven psychological exercises that help calm the brain, body, and emotions during times of stress and anxiety. I have some of my clients do some of these, and I do some of these myself. These exercises are not intended to be a cure all—wham-bam and you're done! However, they do provide significant help and relief. Sometimes we may have to do them several times in a row or several times throughout the day to get the relief we are needing and looking for. Also, this is not an exhaustive list of exercises.

These exercises are *not* listed in order of importance or competence. Also, if you notice the 0–10 beside them, this stands for 0 being ineffective and 10 being very effective in providing relief. The closer a person gets to 10, the more effective the exercise is for them. I put the "0–10" beside each one for the reader to mark the effectiveness the particular exercise has on them. This way the reader has an awareness of what works better for them in providing relief as we know one size doesn't fit all of us all the time because we are different. I would suggest trying each exercise about four times before placing your number next to it. This way your number reflects a body of evidence instead of a singular attempt. You get the idea. Let's begin.

0–10_____ **Deep breathing.** I find this exercise works really well for most of my clients. Therapists may have clients do this slightly differently, adding more or fewer things to do. However, it will work.

Start by getting comfy. You can do this either by sitting in a comfy position or lying down, whatever works better for your particular comfort level. Close your eyes. Pay attention to your muscles. Have the brain communicate to your muscles. to relax. Begin to relax the muscles. Begin to breathe slowly in through the nostrils. Make sure the slow, deep breaths are "from the belly" and not the chest. If it's done correctly, the belly will go out as we inhale and deflate slowly as we exhale. When you inhale, make sure it's slowly and all the way in till you can't take in any more air. Think about how long it takes to slowly inhale. For example, let's say slowly inhaling takes four seconds. Hold your breath for four seconds, and then exhale slowly for four seconds (the same amount of time it took to inhale). But after you hold your breath for four seconds, pucker your lips like you're blowing out a candle. Slowly exhale, breathing out the mouth. Exhale slowly until all the breath is slowly out of your lungs. As you do this, your belly will slowly deflate (go in). After this, repeat these steps about four to six times again, trying to stay relaxed through the whole exercise. After, open your eyes and feel the relaxation in your mind, body, and emotions.

Some may ask, "What are the mechanics of this? Why does this work?" Great question. In short, it tricks the brain by telling it that "all is okay." When we are stressed, anxious, or fearful, our bodies "dump" cortisol in our system, which completely changes our metabolism. High levels for longer periods of time can be

Proven Stress-Relieving Exercises

harmful to us. When we are stressed, anxious, or fearful, we breathe more shallowly without realizing it. When we breathe shallowly, our brain "gets a phone call," and the message is, "Hey, the body is breathing shallowly! There's a reason to be on high alert! Be aware! Be on guard! Something is coming!" Then, the amygdala takes over. When we do the deep-breathing exercise, we are breathing slowly and deeply. This "calls the brain," and the message is "Breaths are slow and deep. Everything is okay. Whew! We can relax. No apparent threat. Let's grab a cup of coffee and relax." So, this tricks the brain into believing that all is well.

Try this exercise about four different times and rate it 0–10, with 10 being very effective. If it's a 6 to 7 or above, this will be a good exercise to consider when stress, anxiety, or fear hits.

0–10_____ **Progressive muscle relaxation.** Let's start by getting in a relaxed position. Comfy? Okay, let's begin. You'll start with your facial muscles and slowly work down to your toes, one muscle group at a time. Once the muscle group is scrunched, or tightened, hold it for ten seconds, release it, and then move on to the next muscle group. Start with the forehead by raising the eyebrows. Crinkle the nose. Tighten the jaw. Tighten both shoulders. Tighten both biceps, which should tighten the forearms, too. Tighten both hands and fingers (and thumbs). Tighten chest muscles. Tighten stomach muscles. Tighten buttocks. Tighten thighs. Tighten calves. Scrunch or tighten both feet and toes. Once done, feel the tension that's diminished. Enjoy it for a bit.

"How and why does this work?" Great question. Doing this exercise stresses the muscles and then relaxes them. It works tension out of the already tense muscles. *Ahh.* It tells the brain "all is well."

Try this exercise about four different times and then rate it 0–10. If it's a 6 to 7 or above, it should be a good "go-to" exercise for relaxation.

0–10_____ **Meditation or our "happy place."** Disclaimer: When I refer to meditation, I am *not* referring to New Age meditation or Eastern religion meditation which, in essence, says, "Completely empty the mind." The Bible's form of meditation is to *think about good things*. Think about the goodness and love and presence and works of God. I can add, too, to think about other things that bring relaxation and a sense of meaning. The apostle Paul, under the inspiration of God's Spirit, penned,

Finally, brothers and sisters, whatever is true, whatever is noble, whatever is right, whatever is pure, whatever is lovely, whatever is admirable—if anything is excellent or praiseworthy—think about such things. (Philippians 4:8 NIV)

Here is one example of a personally preferred and desirable meditation for us outdoors/wilderness kind of folks.

Begin by relaxing in a preferred position (sitting or lying down in a comfy position). Close your eyes. Relax. Try to use all your senses. Imagine you are on the long porch of your log cabin home nestled in an open field with a variety of trees, a river next to you and a view of mountains in the distance. It's fall. The colors are coming out. There is a cool, but not too cool, breeze you can feel on your face and arms. You're sipping a hot cup of coffee that's just perfect to the taste and smell. You're rocking slowly back and forth, taking in the fields, trees with color, mountains in the distance, and the sound of the running river in the distance. The sun is just starting to set. What a beautiful orange tint the sky is sharing. A family of deer come slowly

Proven Stress-Relieving Exercises

into the field. They are grazing on the sweet grass in the early evening. They are just close enough to be seen but far enough not to be spooked. As you watch, you get the slight aroma of crisp fall leaves. In your imagination of this happy place, you can feel the relaxation, enjoyment, and awe of our surroundings. You take it in with a thankfulness to God. You don't want to leave the beauty. Now, sense the relaxation in your mind, body, and emotions. Enjoy this before you get going back into life.

Another example is to sit with your eyes closed and in a comfortable position. Use your imagination (no weird stuff, simply your God-given imagination). Picture some candles burning with their flames going. One candle is for the trauma, another candle is for anxiety, another candle for stress—picture as many candles as you need. Now, picture a calm breath blowing out the candle of trauma. In your mind's eye, look at that flame blown out and relax as the smoke dissipates slowly in the air. Next, picture that same gentle breath blowing out the candle of anxiety. Look at that flame that's blown out. See the smoke of the blown-out candle that represents anxiety dissipating into the air. Relax with it being blown out. Next, picture that same breath blowing out the flame of stress. Look at that blown-out candle with a sense of relief as the smoke from the blown-out candle dissipates slowly into the air. You can continue with however many candles you may have. There is no time limit on this process. Feel the relief physically and emotionally.

Another meditation, or using your God-given imagination, is to close your eyes and think of a closed window and the wind howling as it hits that closed window. The wind howls as it hits the barrier. Now, imagine opening that window to where the screen is visible. As the wind hits the opened window, the howling stops because the barrier of the windowpane is no longer there. The wind simply and gracefully passes through the screen and moves on. If you keep your window (mind) closed, the traumatic thoughts will continue to knock at our window. Those thoughts cannot be resolved. If you open the window, allowing those thoughts in, realizing they happened, that it was unfortunate, you accept it happened, and then the thoughts start to "blow in and blow out."

Let's look briefly at one more meditation, again using our imagination. Close your eyes and try to relax. For those of us who grew up with vinyl records (I know, this dates me), picture the record spinning on the player. The needle is placed on the record. The music is playing. The record is spinning, and the needle on the playing record is the trauma memory. You're "hearing" the trauma! Now, calmly picture your hand, or God's hand, gently taking the needle off the record. Now, the record is still spinning, but there is no sound of music. It's quiet. This represents the fact that the trauma memory is still "spinning" in your thoughts; however, because the needle is off the record now, there begins to come a calm/quiet. You, in this moment, are calming yourself and taking the moment back. In your imagination you can hear the quiet - listen to the silence - and let yourself sense the peace. Do this several times if needed.

This works by using your imagination to picture peaceful moments, which releases the "feel good" chemicals in our brain that help us to relax and enjoy.

Try this about four different times. Rate this exercise on a scale 0–10. If it's 6 to 7 or above, this will be a good "go-to" exercise for relaxing.

0–10_____ **Word Puzzles/Search, puzzles, coloring book, etc.** This is pretty self-explanatory. If you enjoy word puzzles or searches, reading, drawing, painting, or coloring books (they have adult ones), this will be a great way to curl up on the couch, a comfy chair, in bed, or in your studio to enjoy the moment. It's a healthy diversion to take a timeout for self-care, self-love, self-kindness (which, men, we need too). We "get lost" for a little while in peaceful enjoyment.

This works, well, by looking at the last sentence: we "get lost" for a little while in peaceful enjoyment. It relaxes the body, which tells the brain "all is well."

0–10_____ **Praying and reading the Bible or other good books.** For those of you who are believers, this helps you focus on your partnership with God in prayer. Prayer is simply *talking with God.* I've heard it said that *prayer is a wish turned Godward.* Prayer is asking for things, worship and praise, praying for others, thanksgiving, reflection, sharing your joys and anxieties, and so many other things you wish to share. You can draw meaning from knowing that God loves you and hears you, Prayer helps you unload your heaviness to God. It helps you vent your feelings as you put them into words or into writing if you have a prayer journal. You can process life through prayer.

Reading the Bible allows you to see God's ways and His heart toward you and what Jesus did for you on the cross and by His resurrection. He is a living Savior, not a dead teacher whose teachings are just carried out. He lives, interacts, leads, comforts, and intercedes for His children, for us. Reading the Bible causes hope and meaning to begin to well up within us. Also, there are many good books, both fiction and nonfiction, that can provide enjoyment and relaxation.

I've read secular articles from doctors who have reported that after surgeries, patients who had faith recovered faster than patients who did not. It seems that having faith helps by allowing us to think about those things which are good, noble, true, and so on. It helps us to rewire the brain toward the positive. Also, we take comfort in looking to *someone* much bigger than ourselves.

Try this about four times, then rate this from 0–10 with 10 being great. If this is a 6 to a 7 or higher, this will be a good relaxation technique.

0–10_____ **Talking to a close family member or a close friend**. This is self-explanatory. Talking is really good therapy, hence the term *talk therapy*. Supportive relationships are some of the best therapies for PTSD/CPTSD. You can honestly share, be listened to, cared about, validated, possibly get an outsider's view when needed (sometimes we just need to talk with no advice given), and process our emotions, and we begin to calm. We've heard people say, "Boy! I needed to get that off my chest! I feel better." Again, it's called talk *therapy*.

This helps by building connection and relationship with a close, caring, trusted human being in the form of a family member or friend. (If possible, it can be helpful to have several or more close and caring individuals to talk to. This way you don't burn out the one person.)

Try this at least four times and rate its effectiveness on a scale from 0–10, with 10 being very effective. If it's a 6 to a 7 or above, this is an effective means of relieving stress and anxiety.

0–10_____ **Journaling**. This has been a Godsend for me. Of course, for journaling to be effective, a person must somewhat enjoy writing. If so, get a journal or a notepad, a pen, and some free time to write, or grab a laptop or a tablet. (You can even make an audio journal if your keyboarding is rough.)

In journaling, let's look at a few unimportant things. Though proper punctuation, sentence structure, and fluidity are important in writing, journaling *isn't* that. Don't worry about these things as those worries will hinder therapeutic writing. Our goal, as I tell my clients, is to write *real and raw*. It has to be honest and honest to God (He knows anyway, and He cares) about the yuck that we are going through on the inside. It's a "no judgment" exercise! Don't judge yourself for the real and raw emotions that you need to feel and to get out. If you do, it's a vicious cycle just like a dog trying to catch its tail. The guilt from your judgement can make you feel worse, so you may not write raw and real because you may feel even more guilt. Then the dynamic of shame visits.

In journaling, or therapeutic writing, how are you feeling? What real and raw emotions are under the surface: anger, unfairness, disgust, bitterness, depression? Are there feelings of hatred, of vengeance, of poor self-worth/esteem/confidence? What "un-Christian" feelings are you trying to deny, hide, or ignore because they "aren't Christian"? To be effective in journaling, or therapeutic writing, you must drop the denying, hiding, and ignoring. You are you, and your real and raw feelings are your feelings.

For those of us who are believers, we have the new covenant heart (Eze. 36:26 NIV). The anger or bitterness or hatred are not *in* our heart, they are things we *feel*. Though we don't like those feelings, which is good not to like, they are not *in* our heart. They are feelings. We don't need to be ashamed of them and deny, hide, or ignore them. They're there for a reason. In fact, the apostle Paul put it this way: "For the word of God is alive and active. Sharper than any double-edged sword, it penetrates even to dividing soul and spirit, joints and marrow; it judges the thoughts and attitudes of the heart" (Heb. 4:12 NIV). It divides or distinguishes between the two, soul and spirit, and joints and marrow. The Greek word for soul is *psuche*, and the Greek word for spirit is *pneuma*. God has the ability to know what are thoughts and emotions, what's our psychology, and what's from the heart. So, we need not be afraid of feeling and expressing ourselves.

Let's go back to the new covenant heart. God said He gives a new heart and a new spirit and He gives His (Holy) Spirit. And God "downloaded" His desires there. God doesn't give defective new hearts. Paul said we are a new creation in Christ (2 Cor. 5:17). He said it was no longer he (Paul) who lived but Christ who lived through him (Gal. 2:20). That's secure. Sure, we are learning and growing. Of course. With this, these passages are true to the core, too.

Paul said in Romans 12:2 to be transformed by the renewing of your mind, not the heart but the mind, the way we perceive and think. It's not a heart issue anymore but a thinking and old patterns issue. Paul said that we became obedient from the heart (Rom. 6:17). Obedient from the new covenant heart! So, we're not renewing the heart because it's new, we're renewing the way we think. There's a difference because there's a new covenant.

Now, let's tie all this together with Hebrews 4:12 about God *distinguishing between* soul and spirit, joints and marrow. *He knows the difference!* This is great news! When we're struggling as believers with feelings of disgust, hatred, bitterness, or rage from our PTSD/CPTSD, it's not a heart issue but a thinking issue that affects our emotions. Our hearts don't suddenly become "bad." We're *not* disgust or hatred or bitterness or rage; these emotions are what we are *feeling* due to a trigger that alerted our computer (our brain) that caused feelings to surface and sent our amygdala toward the cockpit.

Proven Stress-Relieving Exercises

Why am I "camping on this"? Because we as believers can deny, hide, and ignore how we are truly feeling because "it's not Christian to feel this way," we're told. I've been a believer for forty-three years at this point and was told, overtly and covertly, that these feelings are negative, and it's not Christian to feel these! Sure, it's not Christian to *act* on these; however, you feel what we feel, especially when PTSD/CPTSD is in the equation. These feelings must be felt and expressed (in healthy ways) and processed. One way is therapeutic writing (or journaling). If we as believers think these feelings are bad and un-Christian, what are we going to do with them? We will deny them, hide them, and ignore them. We won't write them out. But if we understand that these are feelings and not coming from our heart (the true and real us), we will engage in feeling them and writing them in our journal to express, process, and get these feelings out.

The best definition for depression that I've heard is *anger turned inward*. In other words, taking the pain and rage and fear and stuffing them, denying them, hiding them inside. Journaling does the opposite.

At times when I'm angry or triggered and feel like picking a fight with the wife, I'll go to my journal and write real and raw. I'll write out the things I feel like saying to her, really allowing myself to feel the anger and writing the anger out. After two, three, or four pages, I can feel the anger dissipating. My writing is slowing down. My words I'm writing are much less intense. I close my journal and have more clarity if I need to talk to her about it, or sometimes I'm able to let it go. If I need to talk to her, I'm more calm due to getting it out in my journal, and I'm more able to have a productive conversation to problem solve. My bride is thankful.

Rate the journaling exercise from 0–10. If it's a 6 to 7 or above, this may be a good exercise to "put in the ol' tool box" for relief.

0–10_____ **Going to therapy (seeing a therapist).** This may be super helpful. There are certain areas in PTSD/CPTSD that may only be navigated through with a professional therapist. I would suggest finding a therapist who specializes in trauma, grief, and PTSD/CPTSD. Not all therapists do. You don't want a "hard-nosed" therapist when dealing with trauma, grief, and PTSD/CPTSD. You want someone who understands the dynamics of trauma, grief, and PTSD/CPTSD and who knows what modalities to use for long-term benefits. You may want a therapist who is relational (more Rogerian) in their approach, with the ability to navigate you through PTSD/CPTSD with loving and respectful accountability and grace with CBT and CPT.

Also, there is a modality called prolonged exposure therapy (PE). This can work well with PTSD/CPTSD. However, you want a therapist who knows how to use it. With severe trauma, PE can produce a lot of anxiety at first; then, over time, the anxiety dissipates, and you gain more control over the feelings related to the trauma. I've used this on myself at various times (but I work as a psychologist). I wouldn't suggest doing this on your own right away. Work with a trained therapist, then, as they lead to that place, they can have you start to do it on your own.

Eye movement desensitization and reprocessing (EMDR) is a type of therapy used for trauma. Results are positive for a lot of clients who have had EMDR in therapy sessions. You'll want to seek out a therapist who is trained and certified in EMDR. You can explore with our therapist whether EMDR might be

Proven Stress-Relieving Exercises

a good fit. It is important to keep looking until you find a therapist that is a good fit. They are out there.

Therapists may recommend medication. If so, they will refer to a psychiatrist for this.

Rate therapy from 0–10 with 10 being great effectiveness. If it's a 6 to 7 or above, this is pretty effective. If not, maybe look into finding another therapist that gets your rating higher.

0–10_____ **Music.** As William Congreve penned in *The Mourning Bride,* "Music hath charms to soothe a savage beast." This is *not* to say that PTSDers/CPTSDers are "savages." What's your genre? Country, rock, pop, jazz, classical? Find music that is relaxing to your soul. Get comfy. Let's think about your muscles relaxing and the tension going out, and be in the *moment* with the music, the various instruments and how they blend in beautiful harmony. Enjoy a hot cup of coffee, hot tea, an ice-cold Cherry Coke, or whatever the choice of beverage is. Enjoy. (My good buddy Rich loves music. It's good therapy for him, and I love seeing his body language relax when he's in his "music zone.")

Now rate this 0–10. If it's a 6 to 7 or above, this is a good tool that brings relaxation.

0–10_____ **Taste experience.** What? Let me explain. An important thing that we rarely do is *live in the present moment.* We call this *mindfulness.* How many of us, when we eat, actually pause and experience the taste, texture, temperature, and delicious blend of the pasta and cheese and sauce? When we sip our coffee, how many times do we taste the coffee, the blend of cream and a hint of sugar? Do we relish the warm feeling as the coffee goes down into our belly? How many times when we sit in our La-Z-Boy do we actually think about the softness of the chair, the cool feel of the leather, and the feeling of our feet propped up? My guess is rarely because so many of us—myself included—live on autopilot many hours in the day. We exist, but we're not really living in the moment. This is *not* to say this is easy. No. With this, it's a few puzzle pieces toward relaxing, retraining our brain, and eventual healing.

Let's look at a few examples.

When you start feeling triggered, let's try this: A taste test! Grab half a banana, and cut it into pieces. Take a couple slices of an orange. Grab a few strawberries. Then, take maybe six blueberries. Use whatever fruit is in the house. Place it on a plate. Sit in a comfy place. Tell your body to relax. Then, take one piece of the fruit. Begin to chew it. Be present in the moment. Taste the fruit. Feel the texture in your mouth. Taste the sweetness or the tartness. Feel it on your tongue. After swallowing, enjoy the residual taste on the tongue and the sweet—or tart—aftertaste. Next, take a different piece of fruit. Follow the same steps. How does it compare in taste and texture to the prior piece of fruit? Enjoy. Take the next piece of fruit. Follow the same steps until the fruit is gone. This will take you out of autopilot and into the present moment to embrace and enjoy the moment. Again, this is mindfulness. Begin to sense the relaxation, even if it's only a little.

Another example can be this. Take a "feel experience." Get a cotton ball, a piece of sandpaper, a little scoop of jelly or jam, a teaspoon of salt, and a tablespoon of cooking oil. Place them on the table. Sit down and tell your body to relax. Next, pick up the cotton ball. Feel the softness and texture. Rub it with your fingers. Maybe rub it up and down your arm. Be in that moment. Next, pick up the sandpaper. Gently rub it between

Proven Stress-Relieving Exercises

the thumb and index finger. Feel the roughness, the sandiness, the grittiness. Next, rub your fingers in the jelly or jam. Feel the cool and squishy texture. Smell the jelly, and then lick it off your fingers and relish the taste. Is it grape? Is it strawberry? Is it marmalade? How does it compare to the cotton ball? Go to the next, and the next, and so on. Feel that particular item. Feel the difference in each texture. Enjoy the various degrees of how each item feels on your skin and to the touch. This helps you to be in that present moment. *Ahh.*

Rate this exercise from 0–10, with 10 being very effective. If it's a 6 to 7 or above, this may be a good calming exercise to come back to.

0–10_____ **Pet or animal therapy.** Have a pooch, a cat, a fish, or a bird? These little (or big) friends do wonders for our mental health and relaxation. Of course, we have to like animals for this to be effective. Many PTSDers find equine therapy (with horses) to be very helpful. Animals show unconditional love. Pets are not "out to get us." Their love, companionship, and presence make us feel not alone. They don't talk back and give us advice. We don't have to perform for them. According to some medical reports I've read, petting your pet actually helps reduce blood pressure, decrease heart rate, and decrease stress. Find enjoyment in Fido or Fluffy or Brutus. What do you love about your pets? What about them makes you laugh or smile? Watch them as they "beat up" their little toy or roll around with their catnip. Watch them as they enjoy their meal or a treat. Talk to them in your loving and silly "pet voice." Enjoy.

Now, rate this on a scale from 0–10, with 10 being really effective in our relaxing. If it's a 6 to 7 or above, pet or animal therapy will be a good tool to help reduce triggers, anxiety, and fear.

0–10_____ **Hobbies.** What's your hobby? Woodwork? Martial arts? Painting? Drawing? Hiking? Bike riding? Walking? Driving to see different little (or big) towns that you've not been to? Sunrises? Sunsets? Stargazing? These can be relaxing, anxiety-reducing, healthy diversions for you to "keep ahead" of PTSD/CPTSD. These are not denial of PTSD/CPTSD but healthy diversions to relax and be in the moment.

Engage in and embrace some delightful hobby of yours and rate it from 0–10, with 10 being very effective in being helpful. Maybe some hobbies will score higher than others. If it's a 6 to 7 or above, this will be a good "go-to" for us.

0–10_____ **Budget for a little fun here and there.** If you're like my wife and me, you have a budget because money doesn't grow on trees. In your budget, allocate a little of your earnings for some fun, whether it's dinner, a movie, a new shirt, a trip three hours north or south, whatever. It doesn't have to break your finances. It doesn't have to be expensive every time. But try to do something once a week, once every other week, once a month, whatever it may be. Do something fun, enjoyable, meaningful.

Rate the experience 0–10, with 10 being very effective. If it's a 6 to 7 or above, enjoy!

0–10_____ **Intentional exercise.** These can include push-ups, pull-ups, sit-ups, walking, swimming, biking, other forms of cardio, weightlifting, and so on. You don't have to live in the gym or do these three hours straight. You can even do these at home or in your neighborhood. Three times a week is good. This offers you a good diversion for a while, working tension out of your muscles and allowing those "feel good" brain chemicals to do their work. You not only get healthier, but you feel emotionally better, too.

Rate this 0–10, with 10 being great. If it's 6 to 7 or higher, put on your walking shoes!

0–10_____ Eating better, especially cutting out sugar. Now, I'm not a primary care physician. Check with your doctor/nutritionist before making any dietary changes or beginning an exercise program.

I cut out sugar about a year and a half ago. Amazing! My irritability went way down, my thinking became much clearer, my energy went up, and I lost a good amount of weight (in a slower and healthy way). I bought foods with no sugar, no added sugar, or very low sugar. Very little flour went into my belly, too. I had to buy new clothes.

One teaspoon of sugar equals about 4 grams of sugar. Wow! That was a lot of extra irritability for me! Don't get me wrong, I'll have one splurge meal and one splurge dessert a week. That's enjoyable. With this, it's way, way, way less sugar intake than I'd normally have.

Try it out. Give it a month to see how it is. Rate it 0–10, with 10 being great. If it's a 6 to 7 or above, we should be feeling better just down the road.

0–10_____Oxytocin increase and cortisol decrease. Oxytocin is known as the "emotional bonding hormone." In short, it's released during touch. Cortisol is the primary stress hormone. Cortisol is released during stress. High and prolonged stress can be dangerous. We all know that with PTSD/CPTSD, there are high and prolonged periods of stress, especially during triggers. It's good to get the stress down.

I was at a seminar about seven years ago that dealt with stress, anxiety, and panic attacks. The speaker (I cannot recall her name, unfortunately) said that touching ourselves in places that can stimulate certain nerves can help calm us and even get us out of a panic attack fairly quickly. According to the speaker, lightly rubbing the bridge of the nose and forehead, wrapping your arms around yourself (like a hug), and rubbing your shoulders and arms can release oxytocin, which decreases cortisol, and will begin to calm you. The body knows this. I can't recall how many times when I was stressed that I'd automatically start to rub the bridge of my nose and forehead to calm myself. This was before I knew to do that

Try this and rate it 0–10, with 10 being very effective. If it's a 6 to 7 or above, this is a good practice for you to engage in.

0–10_____ **Temperature change.** This is a skill I learned from dialectical behavior therapy (or DBT) in a seminar from its founder, Marsha Linehan. It's part of the T.I.P. (Temperature, Intense exercise, Paced breathing) skill.

First, get a bowl that's large enough to put your face in it. Yes, you heard correctly: your face.

Second, fill the bowl with cold water.

Third, put a bunch of ice cubes in it. Let it sit for a few minutes to get good and cold.

Fourth, hold your breath and place your face in the cold ice water. Don't submerge the ears in it, just the face (chin, cheeks, forehead).

Fifth, stay in the ice water for about twenty-five seconds.

Sixth, take your head out of the bowl of ice water. (Repeat if needed.)

Proven Stress-Relieving Exercises

This is supposed to cool your body temperature to where it affects your emotions and helps you calm from anger, stress, or anxiety.

Try this and rate it from 0–10, with 10 being very effective. If it's a 6 to 7 or above, this may very well be a good "go-to" tool to help in times of anger, stress, or anxiety.

0–10_____ **Support group.** These can help well. When I had a practice in Traverse City, Michigan, I facilitated a veterans support group. These men and women had PTSD from their time in the military, being deployed, and being in war. What a great group of men and women. I always left our group feeling two inches tall. It was *not* because of anything they did wrong; they treated me like royalty. But, honestly, I knew I was among giants and heroes. To hear these men and women—tough men and women—become vulnerable and transparent and share and carry each other was a blessing beyond a blessing.

Try a support group for what may fit your particular trauma. Rate it from 0–10, with 10 being great. If it's a 6 to 7 or above, this will more than likely be a great resource for you.

0–10_____ **Gratitude.** Gratitude is, of course, being thankful and appreciative for the good things (the blessings) you have in your life. Gratitude can be blessings you think about for a few moments, it can be some blessings you write down/journal, or it can be some blessings you speak out loud. These are all great ways you can be appreciative. True gratitude changes the way you think, which starts to change the way you feel. It puts you in the present moment, too, especially if what you appreciate is something in the now.

What are you thankful for? What do you appreciate? Your spouse's humor and attractiveness, your kids and their silly laugh, the fact that your family is alive and healthy? The deer in the field as you watch while sitting on your deck with a hot cup of decaf coffee? The morning sun? The sound of the birds? Your little (or big) house that is your refuge? Your pets and their unconditional love they give you? The fact that you have some money in your savings? Good friends? A drive in the country on a cool fall day? The list can go on and on. This helps balance out the difficulties of life. You're *not* denying life's problems; you're just being thankful and appreciative for the blessings, too.

Maybe write down three things in the morning that you are grateful for and then three things before bed that you are grateful for. What a great way to start and end the day and retrain your brain toward gratefulness. At the end of the week or month, review the items you are thankful for. This cultivates gratitude.

Rate this exercise from 0–10, with 10 being great. If it's a 6 to 7 or above, this may be a good exercise to embrace.

As I have said, this is not an exhaustive list of good psychological and stress relieving exercises. There are many others. Once we try these and get used to using some of these tools, this will get us to the place where we are beginning to learn calming exercises. Now, we can start to go to the next phase of CBT and CPT, which can help retrain the brain to start to look at our events and ourselves differently (hopefully with a more positive bent).

As with any therapy tool, let's give ourselves time and grace. These may take a while. Trauma, triggers, flashbacks, fear, anxiety, feeling chaos, and living on edge—these are all real and valid to feel in post-trauma. Some time and grace will help us in the process.

10

Practical Helps to Get the Kind of Life We Want: Helpful Processing

In this chapter we will look at processing trauma, the way we view ourselves, and the difficult emotions we experience with PTSD/CPTSD. To be fair, some readers may have more intense trauma than others. This in no way judges one person's trauma as a seven and another person's trauma as a ten. Trauma is trauma. Period. It's valid. It matters. No questions asked. What I mean is we are all different. Two people can experience the same trauma, but it may have a different intensity for one than the other. This is *not* due to one's weakness, but personality type, resilience level, how one was taught - or not taught-and varying other individual dynamics at play.

Let's start with the question "What is healing from PTSD/CPTSD?" Does healing mean we will *never* have a memory, *never* have a trigger, *never* feel trauma or anger or anxiety or stress or fear? Or does healing mean that after time of grief, mourning, processing, navigating, and living life the *intensity* of the trauma—and the *feelings* associated with it—become less? Like my good friend Chris Hinterman said, "It's there, but it's no longer the centerpiece of our lives." I believe it's the latter one. Why do I believe it is important to identify this? It's important because the first one will set us up for utter failure! Why? It's because the experience of the trauma is programmed in our brain. It's stored. Now, this isn't doom and gloom; it's a reality and validation, but the reality is *also* that we *can* have post-traumatic growth. We can eventually get on with the business of living again, but with scars. This will not set us up for failure because it's realistic. Remember, we're *not* flawed or broken; we've had trauma hit us between the eyes. Experiencing trauma is *not* a character defect.

Let's do what I call the "cranberry juice exercise." If I must give it more of a professional name, "visual processing exercise." Now, this is *not* a "new" therapy; it's just a simple way to visually process healthy approaches to PTSD/CPTSD that I came up with. This will begin to help process trauma and situations, or it will continue to help process, depending where we are at in our individual journey of healing from PTSD/CPTSD. (Note: This exercise may cause anxiety, fear, and discomfort. This is normal. Many times it is good to sit with these uncomfortable feelings so they dissipate. If you're uncomfortable, you may have a loved one present or do this exercise with your therapist.)

Get a big pitcher; however, only fill it with a little juice. We want a lot of extra room to add water later in the exercise. Also, have several (maybe four) small glasses of clear water nearby on the table. Give the juice a name for the trauma. I'm going to use physical abuse.

Write your trauma(s) you have experienced:

_____

_____

_____

_____

Helpful Processing

_____

_____

_____

_____

_____

_____

_____

As you are looking at the juice (representing the trauma), you may feel anxiety, fear, or flashbacks. Reassure yourself this is normal, that you're safe right now, you are okay right now. Maybe do some deep breathing—or other stress-relieving exercise—from the previous chapter.

What are your thoughts and emotions right now?

_____

_____

_____

_____

_____

_____

_____

_____

_____

_____

What sensations are thinking about the trauma causing (e.g., fear, flight response, rapid heartbeat, sounds of trauma, trembling, sweating)? Remember to engage in some of the stress-relieving exercises previously discussed, like deep breathing or meditation. Pause again here and reassure yourself that you are okay, this is normal, you're safe now. This is anxiety producing; however, in the long run, you are breaking the power of the trauma. You are okay and safe; nothing bad is happening right now.

Make a list of any physical symptoms or emotions you're feeling right now:

_____
_____
_____
_____
_____
_____
_____
_____
_____
_____

Next, take a glass of the clear water. This represents healthy actions and beliefs you can begin to take. What is one good, desirable, healthy belief that you can add? For example, *The rape was not my fault. All I did was walk to my car from a friend's house less than a block away. I had to shoot to kill because that's war. I did everything I could to save my mother! I may have frozen, but*

Helpful Processing

that's just the body's response many times to fear. These are all very true beliefs. Pour the clear water representing the healthy belief into the big pitcher with the juice representing your trauma. Notice that the red juice got a little lighter with the clear water added. This is what will happen when you add a good, desirable, healthy belief to your trauma. What belief of yours represented the clear water that was added? (Do this again and again with each good, desirable, healthy belief you can add. Notice that the red juice representing your trauma keeps getting lighter.)

Write some healthy beliefs that you're adding below:

_____
_____
_____
_____
_____
_____
_____
_____
_____
_____

Next, what is a good, desirable, healthy action that you can do to help dilute your feelings about the trauma? Maybe use some of the stress-relieving exercises that worked well, or take a break before you talk when you are angry. Healthy actions come naturally from intentionally adopting a healthy perspective, like realizing that a close relationship with your children is far better than blowing up at them because they left the bedroom light on (or something comparable). Dwell a little more on *what you are* than *what you're not*. An evening walk is better than having that third beer. Depending on the family dynamics, maybe going to Euchre night at brother Bob's this once is better than isolating at home again. Engage more in talking about the trauma, feeling anxious, and using the skills you've found helpful to calm the feelings provoked by the trauma again instead of burying it for the fiftieth time. Look at what you appreciate about your spouse more than what you don't like. Create a thankfulness journal for some of the pure good you have in your life. Give yourself a break, some grace, some self-love, and kindness for the horror you've been through. Say no a little more. Say yes a little more.

What is one action step you can take? Add a clear class of water to that juice for each new action step you can take.

Write your action steps below:

_____
_____
_____
_____
_____
_____
_____
_____
_____
_____

Helpful Processing

Are you noticing how much lighter the juice is getting with all the clear glasses of water being added? This is what adding new, good, desirable, and healthy beliefs and actions will do to your trauma over time. Healthy thoughts and actions dilute the feelings your trauma causes (so to speak) by retraining your brain by developing new neural pathways by processing differently. Healing begins to take place over time.

Again, there's nothing magical about this exercise. It's *not* a new modality or a new therapy. It's *not* a new evidence-based intervention. It's just an easy visual for us to see the trauma represented by the red juice and the new, good, desirable, and healthy beliefs and actions we can start to develop represented by the clear glasses of water that are added to the juice. As we see the juice getting lighter and lighter and lighter in color, we can see how the new, good, desirable, and healthy beliefs and actions can help our trauma "fade" over time. The trauma never goes away. The juice never loses its red hue. However, it fades as each new clear glass of water is added over time. Our trauma can fade, too, through this process we've called post-traumatic growth.

Here's a word picture that can help us process how to get unstuck due to our trauma.

I'm sure a fair number of us have gotten stuck in snow with our cars. Try as we may, our tires keep spinning and spinning and spinning, but our car is going nowhere, hence the expression "spinning your wheels!" This has happened to me a few times.

Why is our tire spinning and spinning but we're going nowhere? It's because we don't have any traction! To get unstuck, we need some traction. In other words, we need something for our tire to grip that takes us from stuck to unstuck. Now, we're moving again.

PTSD/CPTSD is the snow. Our life is represented by the car, stuck, running full throttle but going nowhere. Our spinning tire that's going nowhere is our life that is stuck by PTSD/CPTSD and the same maladaptive coping skills we think will help but don't. What's needed? Traction! Something for our lives to grip that will take us from being stuck to unstuck. What's that? Ready for this? Kitty litter. Kitty litter? Yes, kitty litter. In a real instance of getting stuck in snow or on an icy patch, a good amount of kitty litter sprinkled around the tire and at the edge of the tire can give the tire traction to grip the slipping snow and ice. It can help get you unstuck and get your life moving again.

What are some different coping skills we can use to produce forward motion? Diet, exercise, counseling, therapy, and hobbies are a few. What can you add or remove from your life that will improve how you respond and feel when your trauma looms? For example, instead of six beers after dinner, have two and go for a walk.

What comes to mind?

_____

_____

_____

_____

_____

_____

_____

_____

Helpful Processing

I hope and pray this isn't offensive. I'm *not* meaning to be. I'm *not* trying to minimize anyone's trauma by using processing tools like juice or kitty litter. It's simply a familiar visual and a word picture that can help us process practical approaches, both thoughts and actions, that can help get us from here to there, eventually. That's all. If it was offensive or simplistic to anyone, I offer my heartfelt and sincere apology. Thank you.

As I think about my practice and helping clients get "unstuck" from various places in their lives, here are a few tools that come to mind. Some readers may find some of these fairly helpful.

1. Visit the past to grieve, visit the future to plan, but live most of life in the present moment. Let's find some meaning here and now.
2. Sometimes to get what we want and need for our lives, we have to let something else go.
3. Identify your F.E.A.R. (False Evidence Appearing Real).
4. Stretch a little more than you think you can while being kind to yourself at the same time.
5. If your feet are in two different boats that are drifting in opposite directions, which boat do you need to put the other foot in?
6. Pray, plant seeds, and let Jesus who is in us help us trust God.
7. What does wisdom say?
8. Commitment to what's good and right can make desire a reality.

9. "To live a creative life, we must lose our fear of being wrong." —Joseph Pearce
10. What are our deep, lasting desires within us? (Abandon guarantees and embrace healthy risks regarding them.)
11. Enjoy the little things in life for they truly are big things.
12. Nothing changes if nothing changes.

I know we looked at journaling earlier. This has been a Godsend to me to help me process my thoughts and feelings that seem like a volcano inside of me at times. Though I am far from an artist, some of my journal entries are drawings—okay, stickmen or faces. I'll draw a stickman climbing steep mountains to represent my inner and outer challenges I feel and face in life. I've drawn a stickman on a deserted island with shark fins above the surface of the surrounding water to represent my feelings of isolation and that "things" look like they are against me. I've drawn being on a rowboat in a hurricane with high winds, raging water, lightning, and rain to represent my struggles and confusion and fear. I've drawn myself crossing a high bridge that starts to give way to possibly represent me trying to "get to the other side of life" and God's hand under the breaking bridge to catch me if I fall. I've drawn happy faces, sad and tearful faces, angry faces, confused faces, and numb faces to represent what I was feeling at each of those moments. I've drawn lightning striking me and turning me into dust and ashes to represent what I feel God is doing to me (though I know logically He's not). I've drawn myself in a deep hole with no ladder or no way to get out (to represent my feelings of hopelessness and helplessness).

Point being, journaling—even doodling—is a great way to process "the volcano" of anger or fear or confusion or hopelessness that we're feeling inside of ourselves. Let's do so without

Helpful Processing

guilt, without personal judgment, and without the inner critic shouting at us, "You shouldn't be writing or feeling that!" This is our time of honest evaluation, self-awareness of *us* at that moment, validating *the shit* that has hit us with hurricane force in life. We're creating a "sacred space" for ourselves to be truly loved and feel safe before God, and in the long run, we'll be better for our raw and honest journaling/processing.

What about CBT? It's thinking about what we're thinking about. It's about challenging thoughts that may very well be unhealthy to dwell on for longer periods of time. It's about silencing our inner critic. It's challenging the core beliefs that are dysfunctional. This doesn't mean we have to run around being Positive Pete or Peggy 100 percent of the time. But it also means we don't have to be Negative Nate or Nancy 100 percent of the time either. There is a good balance. Remember, we're retraining our brain to "pave new roads" that our thoughts can "drive down." This affects our lives as thoughts affect our feelings and *how we feel*. Easy? No. It sure wasn't for me. Good? Oh, yes.

I remember my mother dying shortly after a "simple" surgery. I was blindsided! I saw her die in front of me as the doctors and nurses were trying to resuscitate her on the table to no avail. That image haunted me at night! I remember *bargaining* (which is a stage of grief) and telling my wife that *I should have seen the signs that she wasn't doing well! I should have been able to help her! If I had caught it soon enough, maybe she'd still be here! It was partly my fault for not catching that she was declining!* The guilt was enormous! My wife was very compassionate and sensitive toward my grief and mourning (thank you, babe). She gently kept reassuring me, *Honey, you couldn't have known. You're not a doctor. How could you have known she was declining? She looked like she was getting better. If you knew, you would have done something to help her. It wasn't your fault. You did what you knew to do. When you realized she was declining, you told me to call 911. You loved your mom well, and she knew it.* After her consistent reassurance over some time, I started to believe what she was saying. What she was saying was 100 percent true. As I started to believe this, the guilt feelings began to dissipate more and more, though I still grieved and mourned. This helped me challenge untrue beliefs I had, silence my inner critic that saw the opportunity to fillet me to the bone, and to gently place my thinking on what was really true and to start to believe it. Welcome to CBT.

A quick note: This does *not* mean we go around and "correct" hurting people to "see the light" as they are grieving and mourning. No! The Word of God wonderfully proclaims to rejoice with those who rejoice and to weep with those who weep (Rom. 12:15 NJKV). This is God's wisdom and demonstrates His sensitive love toward the grieving. We need to view the context of what's going on. My wife knew that her comments weren't to "fix me" but to comfort me because I was blaming myself harshly. (For further help in this area, please check out my book *Healing the Wounded Spirit, Getting the Permission to Grieve, Finding the Courage to Heal*, published by Xulon Press.)

What are the thoughts or beliefs that haunt us? With truth and kindness toward ourselves, let's begin to take a closer look at what those thoughts and beliefs are and begin to dismantle them with truth and wisdom and kindness toward ourselves. And men, yes, we can use some kindness toward ourselves. Our inner thoughts and wounds and hurts need our kindness. Kindness is strength under control for the good and for our good.

Helpful Processing

What thoughts and beliefs haunt you?

_____
_____
_____
_____
_____
_____
_____
_____
_____

Now, what are some thoughts and beliefs that represent truth, wisdom, and kindness toward you and your traumatic experience? For example, let's say you put as a thought or belief above that you feel what happened was "your fault" and you battle enormous guilt. What can you place in this section that represents truth, wisdom, and kindness? You can put the real reason it *wasn't* your fault (like my wife kindly shared with me).

Write down one truth, one piece of wisdom, and one kindness toward yourself.

_____
_____
_____
_____

_____

_____

_____

_____

_____

If you don't mind me saying, I would look over this second question in the days, weeks, and months ahead to provide the reassurance during triggers and the flare ups of that doggone inner critic.

Another means that can help us process is talking to a close friend, a close family member, and a professional therapist who specializes in grief, trauma, and PTSD/CPTSD. The people closest to us have a big heart, two great listening ears, and the ability to "see from outside the circle" and help us process with truth, wisdom, and kindness. A good support group can help with this as well. There are some good YouTube videos available too that deal with helping us process things we may be having trouble with.

I hope some of this is helpful. It definitely can be. If we're doing some of these things, if we're finding positive, healthy thoughts and actions that help us move forward, great. Let's simply continue in them and maybe add other means we may not have implemented yet. I haven't gone into greater detail on some of the areas I've mentioned because these are starting points that maybe need to be continued and followed up in therapy. A one-on-one therapeutic relationship with a therapist who "clicks" for us is an awesome puzzle piece to our therapeutic picture of healing.

11

Practical Helps to Get the Kind of Life We Want: Facing Giants, Beginning to Heal

What are "our giants," the ones we face every day or nearly every day with PTSD/CPTSD? If we look through the *DSM-5* under PTSD, we'll see many "giants" that we face: hypervigilance, feeling on edge, fear, fight/flight/freeze, anxiety, flashbacks, nightmares, avoidance, anger, withdrawing from others, a hyper startle response, apprehensions, difficulty sleeping, irritability, and the list can go on. These are real "giants."

In the Bible, a young shepherd named David faced a very real giant (physically) named Goliath. Goliath towered greatly over David in height, weight, strength, and skill as a warrior. To the human eye, David was toast! If you will, take your Bible, put this book down, and read this true story for a few moments. The account is in 1 Samuel 17. Try looking at this chapter through the lens of PTSD/CPTSD to draw some comparisons.

Okay. Now that you're back, what do you think? What came to mind reading this? Write your thoughts.

_____

_____

_____

_____

_____

_____

_____

_____

_____

_____

As Goliath towered over young David in height, weight, strength, and skill, don't we feel the same about PTSD/CPTSD? It "towers over us" in height, weight, strength, and skill, too, doesn't it? It may not be a physical person; however, real giants or enemies are more than just physical. PTSD/CPTSD is a mental and emotional giant that affects us physically many times.

Here are some highlights that I picked up from reading this true, historical account that Israel and David faced (looking at it to draw some comparisons to what we face with PTSD/CPTSD).

There was a valley between them (v. 3). Doesn't PTSD/CPTSD create a "valley" between us and what we want to "conquer"? If we're afraid to venture after it, it makes that valley seem even bigger.

Saul and the army of Israel were terrified and deeply shaken at Goliath, his stature, and his threats (v. 11). They experienced the "freeze mode." I get it! Goliath was over nine feet tall (v. 4). Part of his uniform weighed 125 pounds (v.5). The rest of his uniform weighed more. His spearhead alone weighed 15 pounds

Facing Giants, Beginning to Heal

(v. 7). PTSD/CPTSD can cause the strongest of men and women to go into freeze (or flight) mode. It's an enormous giant!

Goliath taunted Israel (v. 8). He ridiculed them, shamed them, intimidated them. Sound familiar? The triggers, the nightmares, the memories of the trauma, the thoughts and feelings of shame, guilt, how we must have failed somehow—how we are *not* men.

David was "nothing special" according to human eyes. He was *just* a shepherd and the youngest at that (v. 14, 15). Who are we to conquer PTSD/CPTSD? We're *just* ordinary men and women. We're not superhuman. We're limited. And it's okay.

David left his familiar surroundings for a while to set out on a journey to take gifts to his brothers (v. 20). With PTSD/CPTSD, we gravitate to the familiar, don't we? Nothing wrong with this for a season until we get acclimated. Then, at times it's both good and healthy for us to leave the familiar for a while and take that journey toward the trauma. This is part of therapy.

Then Israel experienced the "flight mode" (v. 24). All they could see was Goliath's "bigness" (v. 25). Again, I get it! PTSD/CPTSD is big! It's huge! It's intimidating! It's scary!

David inquires what the reward is for slaying the giant (v. 26). Yes, there is a reward in conquering PTSD/CPTSD. We get our lives back. Sure, there are battle scars and wounds. With this, we still get our lives back to a good degree.

David was misunderstood by one of his brothers and falsely accused (v. 28). We will be, too, at times. People who don't have PTSD/CPTSD won't fully get it, unfortunately. Some will try to understand and be compassionate, and some won't.

David respectfully stood up for himself, then walked away from his brother (v. 29). Sometimes, that's all we can do:

respectfully stand up for ourselves so we're not abused and then walk away with honor.

David chose to face the enemy (v. 32). At some point, we will need to face our enemy (PTSD/CPTSD). Long-term avoidance is *not* the answer.

David's critic (v. 33), Saul, knew that in the natural, David was toast! "Don't be ridiculous! There's no way you can fight this Philistine and possibly win! You're only a boy, and he's been a man of war since his youth" (NLT). We may not have physical critics; however, I guarantee you, we will have one big inner critic: our own inner voice telling us how we can't do it!

David validated himself and remembered past victories (v. 34–36). This gave him some assurance that this giant could be the same. Sometimes we just have to recall difficult times that we made it through and let that empower us to face our giants.

David had faith in his God (v. 37). God will do through us what we cannot do by ourselves. There are different times I didn't know how I did it. I knew Someone Else was doing it through me!

David tried Saul's armor (Saul's way), but it didn't fit David. David couldn't wear it (v. 38, 39). Most everybody is going to have an opinion of "what we should do." Some will be wise, loving advice. Some advice is not going to fit—it's not for us, and we will incur harm if we "wear it." Be discerning.

David gathered the tools (stones and sling) that worked for him, that fit him (v. 40). Then, David engaged in the fight (v. 41). What works for us? What doesn't? This self-awareness will help the tools that are effective for us. Then, we can start toward our giant(s).

Goliath's continued intimidation (v. 42–44). Our PTSD/CPTSD will have a voice of its own intimidating us and

Facing Giants, Beginning to Heal

telling us how inefficient we are. We will probably believe it (for a while).

David knew he was not alone in this fight (v. 45–47). As believers in Jesus Christ, we are not alone in our fight with our giants. Yes, we question, we feel alone at times, we feel ourselves sinking and losing touch. Very normal. With this, we are truly never alone. Like I said, we have someone in us doing what we cannot do in and of ourselves.

Goliath moved closer, and David engaged him in the fight (v. 48). PTSD/CPTSD will "move closer" to attack. Believe it. Expect it. Accept it. It's normal. We aren't doing anything wrong. With this, as David did with Goliath, it benefits us in the long run to move toward it, to engage it, to feel it, to weep over it, to get angry about it, to talk about it, to journal it, to engage in stress-relieving exercises, and to process it. Our therapist can help us do this, too.

David used his tools, his stone and sling (v. 49 a). Let's intentionally use the tools we have learned and are learning to win over PTSD/CPTSD. We can't eventually win if we deny the giant. Tools left in the toolbox won't help.

David won over Goliath (v. 49 b–54). Let's look at this for us as post-traumatic growth.

David came before the commander (Saul) with Goliath's head still in his hand (v. 57). Even though we can win over PTSD/CPTSD (post-traumatic growth), we'll still "have Goliath's head in our hand." In other words, we'll still carry "our giant's head," or some PTSD/CPTSD, with us in life. We don't have to carry "Goliath's whole body"; however, we may carry "his head" or the residue or scars with us, which is way better than Goliath's whole body. This is to show how we won't be able to "just get over" the trauma(s) and PTSD/CPTSD.

This doesn't promote hopelessness, I pray, but offers validation and a sense of normalcy. We can have beautiful post-traumatic growth and some awesome healing; with this, the trauma will always be with us to a degree—in the "head" and not the "whole body," anyway.

Boy, I wish I could have a conversation with all of you to see what you gathered from this true and historical account. I bet you drew some great comparisons that I may have missed.

I'd like to simply focus on four of our giants that we face from PTSD/CPTSD. Let's look at shame, guilt, fear, and "the new normal."

I've heard it said that shame is probably the number one foundation to most mental health / emotional challenges. With nearly two decades of being in private practice, I would have to say that I agree.

Shame manifests itself in our PTSD/CPTSD. First, let's distinguish the difference between shame and remorse. Remorse is being sorrowful for *what we did* that hurt someone. This *is* good and healthy. On the other side of the coin, shame is being appalled at *who we are*. Shame attacks us in our personhood. It attacks who we are as an individual. This is *not* healthy, *not* needed, and *not* good. Shame is generally initiated by the narrative we believe that comes from the voices from without (other people) or the voices from within (our very own inner critic). We can be our worst critic many times over.

We can feel shame because *maybe my dress was a little too short, and maybe that's why I was raped.* Or *If only I didn't shoot my gun too quickly, maybe he would have put his down.* Or *If I would have called my mother earlier that day, I would have picked up that she was confused.* Or *If I would have stayed home that day, I wouldn't have gotten into that accident, and that poor man would still be alive.* Or *If I hadn't gone for that evening walk, I wouldn't have been robbed and beaten by those three guys.* Or *If only I would have taken that other job six months ago instead of this one, maybe I wouldn't have gotten laid off indefinitely and lost nearly everything.*

Can you see the *ifs* and *maybes*? We use *ifs* and *maybes* because we are not sure. There's no concrete way to know; however, we look at situation(s) like the examples above and make them concrete, certain that a different outcome *would* have happened. Therefore, due to this subconscious narrative, shame builds in us, and we blame, despise, and loathe ourselves, *who we are* as a person. It's imperative to look at *ifs* and *maybes* in the reality of what they are, which is *non concrete* hypotheticals, only *possibilities* at most. This helps our narrative and gives us some grace and self-kindness that we desperately need in our post-trauma(s). This greatly decreases the shame monster. This is one monster under the bed that needs taming.

What's the shame you're feeling and experiencing?

_____
_____
_____
_____
_____
_____
_____
_____
_____

In what ways can you begin to change your narrative toward some grace and self-kindness?

_____

_____

_____

_____

_____

_____

_____

_____

_____

_____

Regarding guilt, we're going to get different opinions. One group says it's good because it's being sorry for what we have done. Another group says it's not good because it attacks our personhood. They continue to say that *remorse* is a better word to use. Who's right? Maybe they're both saying the same thing, in essence. I like the word *remorse* better.

Guilt, according to my profession, has two labels: *appropriate guilt* and *inappropriate guilt*. As suggested, one is warranted, and one is not. For the sake of my OCD and being a word person, let's use the phrasings *appropriate remorse* and *inappropriate remorse*. Thanks.

An example of appropriate remorse would be remorse for *purposefully* driving over our neighbor's foot with our SUV because he made us mad. Right after that, we realize what a dumb and unwise thing that was to do! We apologize and make things right because you have and sense *appropriate remorse*. It's warranted to be remorseful even if he is a massive jerk.

An example of remorse that's *not* appropriate would be a similar example. We *accidentally* run over our neighbor's foot with our SUV. We're not mad at him, we like him; however, we didn't see him walking up to our vehicle as we were backing out, and we accidentally ran over his foot. Of course, we are going to have and feel remorse. We will apologize, let him know it was an accident, and we'll see how we can help. Good. Where it becomes *inappropriate remorse* is when you stew on our sorrow regarding it for days and weeks. We blame ourselves. Our narrative is *how stupid and incompetent we are!* We lose sleep and appetite. It becomes dysfunctional. This is all for something we didn't mean to do. Sure, sorrow about it being an accident is good, but long-term sorrow and blaming ourselves and punishing ourselves is *not good*.

Hence, the difference between the two.

If this book was purchased or given as a gift to be read, there's a good chance the reader of this book has suffered deep trauma(s). I'm sure it's way more traumatic than the fictional examples I gave above with the appropriate and inappropriate remorse. Because of this, I want to be wise and sensitive in how I proceed.

Someone reading this book is way more than likely reading it because they had a trauma that affected them deeply. The reader has remorse. Why? Because they are a human being with healthy feelings and a healthy mindset, and they're not narcissistic. Many of us may feel we dropped the ball in not acting fast enough, being brave enough, not noticing soon enough, overlooking something, anything. Maybe part of our trauma is that this affected someone we loved deeply. *If it wasn't for us, maybe they'd still be here* is the demon we battle in our mind. So, yes, I get it: inappropriate guilt or remorse is something we battle, and knowing the difference between appropriate and inappropriate remorse isn't going to cause us to jump up and say, "Hallelujah! I'm healed of these feelings!"

If there is a moral injury, this can be even more difficult. A moral injury is when an individual feels their conscience, beliefs, moral compass or values are violated when they have taken part in or witnessed an event that goes against what they value. Combat veterans and law enforcement men and women can be particularly susceptible to this as they protect their lives, the lives of others or follow certain orders.

Let me share a true story of what happened to me at sixteen years old, and beyond, to help illustrate the above.

My parents were divorced when I was maybe three or four years old. One night I went to bed with dad there, and the next morning—and ten years later—he was gone. My mom divorced him because he was abusive when he was intoxicated, and he went away to prison for some decisions he made in life.

One day we got a call that "Earl's out of prison, and he'd like to see little Earl." I was fourteen years old. I remember going over to my cousin's home, with other visitors there, to see him. It felt so odd. I met a man who I kind of remembered but hadn't seen or heard from in more than ten years, and now here he was again. It was sweet and uncomfortable at the same time.

After that, we saw more of him. It was cool to have a dad again. He and my mom got back together, but they didn't remarry. Life went on. However, turbulence happened. It got rough and bumpy. It got hard and difficult. There was alcohol

Facing Giants, Beginning to Heal

and some drugs and physical abuse toward my mom again. Then it got better. Then it got bad.

As a sixteen-year-old young man at this point, I was frazzled with the ups and downs, good and traumatizing, here one day and gone the next, laughing one moment and on the run the next. Whew!

One Saturday my dad came over—because he lived with my grandma—and asked if I would help him mow the lawn at Grandma's house. As I thought for a moment, all the ups and downs, good and traumatizing, here one day and gone the next, laughing one moment and on the run the next, came to a head. I said *no*. Later that day my dad died of a heart attack (his second one) in my grandma's driveway. I got the news later that day when I got home from a friend's house. (We didn't have cell phones then.)

For twenty years after that, I carried the guilt or remorse that *if I had been there, my dad may not have died! I could have cut the grass, and he maybe would have lived! Or I could have called 911 soon enough if I was there! It was my fault because I told him no!* This was my narrative for twenty years!

My then therapist asked me what carrying this was like. I said it was like carrying a large canoe over the top of my head for twenty years. Then she asked me a question that began to change my narrative, and I began to "put the canoe down." She said, "Earl, what if you had known that your dad was going to have a heart attack that day? What would you have done?" It didn't even take me a second to say, "I would have gone and been right there to do what I could." She said, "Exactly! You didn't go because you didn't know." Right then the light bulb came on for me: *I didn't know, and that's why I didn't go. If I had known, I would have gone.* It wasn't my fault after all. Was I remorseful? Yes. But my inappropriate remorse—that his heart attack was *my fault*—began to quickly fade at that point.

Can you identify your inappropriate guilt or inappropriate remorse?

_____
_____
_____
_____
_____
_____
_____
_____
_____

How can you begin to change your narrative toward some grace and self-kindness?

_____
_____
_____
_____
_____
_____

Facing Giants, Beginning to Heal

Fear is another big monster that's under our bed! As I mentioned earlier, the brain does not distinguish between real threat (which produces fear) and perceived threat (which also produces fear). Threat is a threat to the brain, which ignites the fight/flight/freeze response. So, one fair help in dealing with PTSD/CPTSD is being able to intentionally identify our fear or F.E.A.R. (**F**alse **E**vidence **A**ppearing **R**eal). Some fears are real, while some are false. Even with false evidence appearing real, our feelings are valid. They are important and matter. We do want to identify the false evidence appearing real, however, so we are two steps ahead of PTSD/CPTSD and their triggers.

In 2008, the economy crashed, and many, including myself, lost their jobs, couldn't find work, and had to rely on unemployment benefits, which weren't much. Not only was this a significant hit in my life, but I had about five other significant issues hit my life as well. I called this *financial PTSD!* This lasted about two years for me.

Press the fast-forward button. A few years beyond this my wife and I, doing well financially, were in various restaurants as we went out once a week for date nights. For a fair amount of time, at different restaurants, I would anxiously scan over the menu many times, trying to find the least expensive thing on the list that I liked. My heart rate would speed up, I felt tense, I felt worry and anxiety, I felt as if I was back in 2008–2010 emotionally. In this situation, I didn't know the acronym F.E.A.R. (**F**alse **E**vidence **A**ppearing **R**eal). I wasn't aware of the amygdala hijack either. (Not that knowing these is a cure all. However, knowing them would have put me two steps ahead of PTSD/CPTSD.) So, my fear of 2008–2010 gave me a false fear several years later that caused me to anxiously scan the menu looking for the least expensive item.

We are going to have and experience false fears with PTSD/CPTSD. *If I get married again, he could beat me! If I go out after dark, I could get jumped! If I open up, it'll be used against me! If I take this risk, I'll utterly fail! If someone trusts me again, I'll let them down, so I'll keep to myself! If I do that activity, I'll have another heart attack and maybe die this time, so I won't do it!* On and on the beliefs go. Sure, we want to be wise. We want to use wisdom. Equally, we don't want to give in to the F.E.A.R. either. Because it happened then doesn't mean it will now. Are we safe now? Are we in a better setting now? If yes, then let's navigate through the F.E.A.R. We want to stay safe with truth, not with what's false.

Identify your fears.

_____

_____

_____

_____

_____

_____

_____

Facing Giants, Beginning to Heal

_____

_____

_____

_____

Now, out of these fears, identify your F.E.A.R. (false evidence appearing real)?

_____

_____

_____

_____

_____

_____

_____

What are you going to do about the F.E.A.R.?

_____

_____

_____

_____

_____

_____

_____

_____

_____

_____

_____

Before moving on from fear, let me say that this is one of the biggies! Fear paralyzes us. It creates the fight/flight/freeze states. Fear is a shadow to flashbacks. When we have a flashback, fear is right there, too.

The typical go-to coping method to fear is to avoid it. *Don't let the sucker near us!* I get it. It's too hard, and it's too difficult, and it's too much work to face it at times when we need to. Here's the truth though: it's hard, difficult, and too much work to avoid it and keep it buried, too. It's difficult work either way. If it's difficult work either way, why not get the healthiest benefit from the work we do? Let's face it when needed. Over a little time, we'll see that we're facing it more and more.

Like many of you, I too avoided those memories—those conversations, those parts of town, some of those people who reminded me of the trauma (or even very uncomfortable times in my life that may not have necessarily been a trauma). Why? They're uncomfortable man! I noticed though, as I took "baby steps" toward thinking some about the memories and began having some of those conversations and going to those parts of town, sometimes I was able to do so a little more, and a little more, and a little more. Conversely, avoiding those areas could make one "stuck" for a longer period of time. Presently, my intensity of the fears/memories are a zero to a two on the intensity scale. That's great! Now, it took a while to get there; however, I did so on a regular basis. This helped break its power over me.

I say this not to toot my own horn but to show that post-traumatic growth, and some hope, can happen. It takes time, effort, discomfort, reframing, reengaging, and living again (with some scars, yes).

Finally, let's explore our new normal. I dislike this term because *I want a lot of my old normal!* After trauma, however, we have a *new normal:* a normal with memories, a normal with scars, a normal that scans the parking lot before we venture into it, a normal that doesn't trust as easily, a normal that sets boundaries more quickly, a normal that calculates risks more, a normal that double checks the locks on the doors before we go to bed, a normal that gives our kids extra kisses and hugs at bedtime, a normal that says, "I love you," when parting company when this didn't happen as much before, a normal that has a CPL (concealed pistol license), or a normal that has taken self-defense classes or practices martial arts. We get the idea.

Here's a news flash: these new normals *aren't all bad* things! Yes, the memories and fears and scars stink! With this, there's a lot of good that the new normal produces. (Plus, over time, the memories and fears and scars become manageable with therapy and work.)

One of my new normals, after a very traumatic financial event in my life, was that I started thanking God at mealtime *for providing me with the money to purchase this food.* I *never* prayed that way before! Oh, I thanked God for my food, which was great. But now, my thanking goes further to thanking Him *for the money earned* to be able to buy my food. Did God *cause the trauma* to *make me more thankful?* Some would say yes. I say *absolutely not.* Jesus said that in this world we would have tribulation (John 16:33 NIV). My deeper thankfulness came from something that's already in the world that we will face at times—hardships—and God's eventual provision that helped me through those times.

The growth takes many forms. We are wiser. We are more prepared. We are more thankful. We are more sensitive to the trauma of others. We are less judgmental. We are better givers. We are more tactful in our response. We are more kind (strength with control). We set quicker boundaries. We know how to defend ourselves. We are more attuned parents. The list goes on. Some may say, "Earl, I'm sure not any of those yet!" That's okay. Many of us weren't either. But we journeyed there. So will you, my friend.

Can you identify your new normal?

_____

_____

_____

_____

_____

_____

_____

_____

_____

_____

Facing Giants, Beginning to Heal

Can you identify some of the positive aspects that come with your new normal?

_____
_____
_____
_____
_____
_____
_____
_____
_____

As we have seen, there are great benefits in facing our giant and doing the battle to get our lives back. No, it isn't easy, but it's good. Without this, the monster stays under the bed. It may be quiet for a while; however, it will shake our bed, wake us up, and knock us off our bed onto the floor. Then, it will return to being quiet for a while. It needs to go. The good news is that we can get the monster out from under there—eventually.

Conclusion

Final Comments

As you can see, this is *not* an "Everything You Need to Know about PTSD/CPTSD" book. There are more things we could add. However, it would become a thick textbook, and that would probably defeat the purpose because few would read it. Plus, I'm not that smart!

This is a practical, validating, hands-on book to help fellow PTSD/CPTSD sufferers gain the added tools and find the grace and strength needed to continue in their journey. It's a book of reality, hope, and help. At least this is our goal, wish, and prayer.

I realize I didn't reveal much about my traumas. Part of this was on purpose as this book is not a reveal-all-type book about me. That being said, here is a quick rundown to give you an idea about some of my traumas. My parents were alcoholics. My dad physically abused my mom. I remember my mom and me having to hide outside when my dad was intoxicated, angry, and looking for a fight. I remember my dad taking me ("kidnapping" me) when I was little. My dad served time in prison. I grew up on welfare. My mom would beat me physically and leave marks on my body. She would abandon me and leave me with sitters (sometimes for days on end). When we gave our lives to Christ, my mom became a great mom. However, much damage had been done by then. As an adult, I got MRSA and almost died.

I had thousands of dollars stolen from my account several times. I lost my job during the 2008 crash. I was divorced. My mom died in front of me. There's more; however, I think this "qualifies me" as knowing a little about trauma.

I became irritable and angry. Nothing wrong with this. I ended up burying it for a long time until I couldn't do it anymore. Then, I became hyperaware or hypervigilant. With my traumas, and internalizing it, I felt deep insecurities. I felt "the world" was out to get me. Heck, I felt God was out to get me! This made my irritability and anger more heightened. I was on edge, couldn't truly relax, couldn't enjoy the moment, felt poorly about myself, and missed good opportunities because I was stuck in the past. Sometimes I would rage when I was by myself. Again, perfectly understandable with trauma and PTSD/CPTSD. I wasn't a "bad man" for this. With this, though, I allowed myself to suffer, and some of my relationships suffered as well. This is when PTSD/CPTSD truly works *against us*. My poor wife took the brunt of my irritability and anger to where she, as the Beatles sang about, "had a ticket to ride."

Looking back—with hindsight being 20/20—what have I learned? Would I have done things differently? I've learned and am still learning things. Yes, I would do things differently. This is where we have to be careful to not butcher ourselves and beat ourselves up beyond recognition because we probably did the best we could at the time. So, no butchering but simply reflecting informed by wisdom learned.

I will highlight three things here, though there are more that I would have done differently. After I share, let's reflect on what each reader would have done differently and what can be done now in the present.

Final Comments

One, I would have gotten counseling much sooner. Yes, the psychologist would have gotten counseling from another therapist. Yes, I would have had to swallow my pride and admit that I needed help *too* and that getting that help was a needed journey for me *too*. Don't get me wrong; working as a psychologist, I knew some good things to do to navigate through my traumas, and I was engaging in some of those good things. With this, however, *I* needed someone *I* could talk to who knew good, proven, and kind tools, too. Even Jesus needed *someone else* to help carry His cross.

I'm glad to say that for about two years now I have had my own therapist who has helped me walk through some pretty difficult seasons of my life and given me some kind perspectives. She has helped me relearn the need for some real kindness toward myself. Though I'm still on this journey, my symptoms have gone way down. Thanks, Danielle.

Two, I would have been much more intentional about enjoying the present moments that were good. Now, this doesn't eliminate healthy grieving. I still *needed* that. With this, there were good, cherishable moments that I only enjoyed between 0 and 50 percent because of my traumatic memories. Nothing wrong with traumatic memories. These are *normal*. The balance is, however, being able to intentionally enjoy some of the good, cherishable moments, too. It's *both*.

Looking back, I can pick key moments when I could have intentionally enjoyed those moments or those seasons. Those good and cherishable moments would have been healing for my soul and enjoyment to my CPTSD bones. I can't get those moments back. They're gone forever. Now, should I beat myself up for missing those moments? No way. Now, I can learn from that and intentionally enjoy new good and cherishable moments that come along. They are God's new gifts to bring healing to my soul and enjoyment to my CPTSD bones.

Three, I would have realized that my anger affects others. I *knew* about this, but I didn't *know* this for me. It's okay to be and feel angry. It's one of those God-given emotions that are to be used, too. Some would do well to be able to express their anger in more healthy ways. My problem was with the second half: expressing my anger *in healthy ways*. I wasn't a monster. However, I wasn't easy to live with either. My wife was walking on egg shells for a long time. My irritability and anger were over the smallest stuff. I was hurting. *Nothing wrong* with this. It's just that wisdom realizes there are others in my circle who are affected, too. That's all. I finally saw how my anger was affecting her. It broke my heart, and I had a change of thinking and direction. Am I perfect at dealing with my anger? Probably not. About 95 percent better? I believe so.

With these three lessons learned, it's a continuous journey for me.

What about you? What are some lessons learned as you look back? What do you think you'd do differently if you could?

_____

_____

_____

_____

_____

_____

_____

Final Comments

I like how Dr. Andrew Farley puts it: "God is not in love with some future version of you. He's in love with you now." Same idea: God is not considering us a "better us" when we finally get healed. He's considering us to be a "good us" now as we're on our way toward healing.

Let's continue to learn that how we view things—like the above—and how we talk to ourselves goes a long way with positive or negative repercussions.

Annalise's and my prayer for you is taken from Ephesians 3:

> *I pray that out of his glorious riches he may strengthen you with power through his Spirit in your inner being, so that Christ may dwell in your hearts through faith. And I pray that you, being rooted and established through love, may have power, together with all the Lord's holy people, to grasp how wide and long and high and deep is the love of Christ, and to know this love that surpasses knowledge–that you may be filled to the measure of all the fullness of God.* (Ephesians 3:16–19 NIV)

Thank you.

Authors' Biographies

Annalise

I feel that a bio would be redundant at this point. I have opened my life to you, the reader, far more than a quick bio could ever accomplish. I prefer to be the person in the crowd that no one notices. It's easier that way. I trust that those reading this book will get a sense of knowing me without a bio. At some point, I may come out of my anonymity. Names have been changed to protect our privacy.

Earl

I received my bachelor's degree from Great Lakes Christian College in Lansing, Michigan, and my master's degree in counseling psychology from Michigan Theological Seminary (now Moody Theological Seminary) in Plymouth, Michigan. I've had the privilege of being in ministry for about forty years, which includes volunteering, pastoring, and serving as a hospice chaplain. I've been an adjunct professor at Baker College and Spring Arbor University. I've been in private practice for nearly two decades at this point. God is helping me be transparent and vulnerable with the traumas I have suffered to help fellow sufferers as well.

www.ingramcontent.com/pod-product-compliance
Lightning Source LLC
Chambersburg PA
CBHW070520090125
20085CB00006B/105